Stop Knee Bursitis Pain

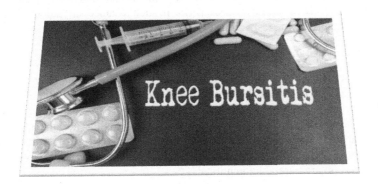

Prepatellar, Pes Anserine, Infrapatellar and
Suprapatellar Knee Bursitis

Symptoms, causes, exercises, treatment, surgery, injections,
diet, remedies, and more..

Graham Wright, MPhil, Ph.D.

About the Author

Graham Wright holds a Ph.D. from Imperial College in London, UK and has extensive research experience spanning over 20 years in academic and applied research institutions. Graham's passion and area of expertise is conducting research on the various conditions of the musculoskeletal system and sharing his findings, knowledge and enthusiasm through his informative medical books.

After reading a news article on the fast-growing incidence rates of Knee Bursitis, he searched online and realised that the information targeted specifically to Knee Bursitis in the public domain is really scarce. He then decided to write a book on this subject to help millions of people suffering from the condition worldwide. He conducted thorough research on the entire published literature and distilled all the information he collected in these pages in an easy-to-read and comprehensible style.

In a Nutshell

Stop Knee Bursitis Pain provides you with all the tools and methods you will need to completely alleviate your Knee Bursitis pain and take back control of your life.

The author, Graham Wright, MPhil, Ph.D., gives you all the required background on Knee Bursitis, while placing the main emphasis of the book on the treatment of the condition. Though this publication is based on all the latest medical research, the author assumes no medical background for the reader and presents all topics in easy-to-grasp everyday language.

This book is the Ultimate Guide to becoming an expert on your Knee Bursitis condition and it is packed with sound advice and tips on how to finally end your knee bursitis pain. So, please don't wait and read on.

Contents

Introduction

Bursitis is an inflammation of the bursae. Bursae are fluid-filled sacs that are situated around joints and tendons throughout the body. Their purpose is to reduce friction from movement and provide a cushion between bones, tendons, muscles and skin. Bursitis can develop in any joint area of the body.

Knee bursitis can afflict one or both knees. Common symptoms include pain and possible swelling of the affected knee. Patients can find it almost impossible to stand, walk or even lie on the side of the affected knee due to swelling and inflammation.

Pain is usually directly over the inflamed bursae, and the patient can find the motion of the joint very painful. Knee bursitis limits the patient's ability to walk because of the knee motion restriction. Inflammation in the bursae causes pain in the knee joint and the surrounding muscles. All bursitis is not contagious, and it is also not hereditary. Patients can become prone to bursitis because of underlying health or lifestyle conditions, but bursitis does not necessarily reoccur. There are different types of knee bursitis, and knee bursitis can occur in children through to the elderly. Knee bursitis is not a selective disease.

Certain existing health conditions can make patients more susceptible to bursitis as a secondary condition. Common existing health triggers include previous injury from a fall, gout and forms of arthritis. Lifestyle can also trigger bursitis. All of these are discussed in greater depth in later chapters. This book is not written for readers looking for scientific facts on knee bursitis, and it is not intended for academic purposes. It approaches knee bursitis with empathy and understanding. Written in easy to read language, it explains medical terms and gives in-depth information to knee bursitis sufferers. It covers all types of knee bursitis from early onset through diagnosis, treatment, management and healing. It also covers holistic treatments and recommended dietary changes.

Chapter 1: What is Knee Bursitis?

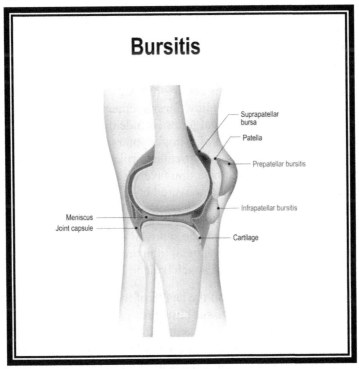

The word "Bursitis" refers to an inflammation of any of the bursae in the body. Bursae are tiny sacs filled with synovial fluid and located at joints and tendons throughout the body. The primary function of bursae is to provide a sort of cushion between the bones, tendons, and the surrounding skin to prevent the harmful effect of friction – wear and tear. Bursitis can develop at any of the bursae in the body.

Knee bursitis occurs when any of the bursae of the knee becomes inflamed. It could affect one or both knees. Common symptoms of the condition include pain and swelling of the affected area. When knee bursitis occurs, it could cause discomfort, affect the mobility of the patient and in severe cases, it could be fatal if the problem is further compounded by the presence of infection.

There are various treatment methods for knee bursitis – ranging from natural treatment to physical therapy, surgical intervention, alternative medicine, exercise and dieting. The severity of the condition will determine which method will be most appropriate.

1.1 Decoding Bursitis

Before we can understand bursitis, we must understand the bursae and their role in the human body. As mentioned in the introduction, bursae are fluid-filled sacs that are situated around joints and tendons throughout the human body.

An adult human body contains about 206 bones and 300 joints. Most joints are synovial joints that allow for movement and bursae are found around synovial joints. Synovial joints include the hips, knees, elbows, fingers and toes. The surfaces of synovial joints are covered with a thin layer of very strong and smooth articular cartilage. The bones that meet to form a joint are separated by a thin layer of synovial fluid that also lubricates, and the two cartilage-covered bone surfaces.

The joint surface is encapsulated by a thin synovial membrane that produces synovial fluid. Behind the synovial is a stringer sub-synovial membrane. Also, around the synovial joint are tendons that attach muscle to bone, ligaments that attach bone to bone and bursae.

Healthy synovial joints rely on the health of the soft tissue structures around them just as the soft tissue structures rely on the health of the bone in the joint. For example, a damaged ligament can cause a joint to become unaligned, and that can eventually lead to joint degeneration and osteoarthritis, which in turn can lead to inflammation of the bursae. It is important to note that all synovial joints are susceptible to arthritis, which in the long term can encourage bursitis.

Healthy synovial joints move together with little or no friction, because they are protected by healthy articular cartilage, synovial fluid and bursae. A healthy synovial joint motion is easy and without any pain.

Understanding Bursae

Bursae are like lubricated pads that are to be found at points of contact and potential friction between bones and the surrounding soft tissue, including ligaments, muscles, skin and tendons. Bursae are situated between bone and the contrasting surface.

In appearance, bursae are thin lubricated pads containing a few drops each of synovial fluid that are wedged between bone surface and any contracting surface.

Some bursae facts include:

- Healthy bursae are thin flat pads measuring no more than about 1.5 inches or 4 centimetres in diameter and about 0.10 of an inch or a few millimetres in thickness
- Each bursa differs in size depending on where it is located in the body
- Some bursae are buried deep with muscle and other soft tissue, while others are situated just below the skin surface
- An adult has about 160 bursae located throughout the body
- Certain bursae are present at birth, while others develop as a result of friction as the body becomes more mobile
- Bursae can develop spontaneously and be unique to an individual in areas of constant friction
- Any abnormal bone formation can result in bursa developing to protect the area

Each bursa is made up of a synovial membrane sac, or synovium, and filled with synovial fluid. The synovium produces the synovial fluid content contained in each bursa, and the synovium is semi-permeable. Synovial fluid is not static, it passes through the walls of the synovium, and other components flow in to and out of the bursae. This transferal of fluid and components in and out allows the bursae to heal if they become inflamed, infected or injured. For example, a bursa can become filled with blood for one of many reasons, and the semipermeable membrane of the synovium allows the blood to drain out. Synovial fluid is clear and viscous. It looks like and has a similar texture to egg white.

Synovial fluid also aids in the nutrition of the articular cartilage that covers the synovial joint surfaces. It acts as a transference medium for nutritional substances. Within the synovium, there are two types of lining cells as well as antigen presenting cells known as dendritic and mast cells that reside in a matrix. The matrix is rich in alpha-1 type I collagen and proteoglycans. Synovial tissue within the synovium contains fat and lymphatic cells, fenestrated microvessels, nerve fibres derived from the capsule and periarticular tissues.

What is Bursitis?

Bursitis occurs as result of the synovial membrane of a bursa becoming inflamed. The inflammation causes the synovium walls to thicken and produces excess synovial fluid, and that causes the bursa to begin swelling. There are many causes of inflammation in the bursae, including injury, excessive friction and infection. An infected bursa will eventually begin filling with pus. Underlying skeletal health conditions like arthritis can also cause bursae to become inflamed.

Bursitis most commonly occurs in the elbows, hips, knees and shoulders, but can also occur in the ankles, buttocks, toes and wrists. It can take anywhere from a few weeks to a few months for bursitis to heal completely, but if there is an underlying health issue like arthritis or a bone or ligament abnormality, bursitis can persist.

Bursae can rupture if the inflammation causes excessive swelling. This can be addressed through surgical removal of the affected bursa. Also, in instances of persistent bursitis that does not abate or respond to treatment doctors might recommend surgical removal. Most joints are unaffected by the removal of bursae and can function without them. Opting for surgical removal of bursae is usually a last resort after other treatments and options have been exhausted. In some instances, a new healthy bursa can redevelop. If this happens, and underlying health issues have been successfully addressed, bursitis might not reoccur.

Inflammation of any bursa can develop slowly or suddenly, depending on what has caused it. Inflammation is a natural part of the body's defence mechanisms against invasion by bacteria, viruses and other foreign bodies. Inflammation is also how the body tries to heal itself after injury and to repair damaged tissue. In the case of bursitis, once the body senses injury a biochemical process is triggered that releases proteins called cytokines. These proteins act as a crisis signal to the body's immune system, hormones and other nutrients which converge on the area in an attempt to repair the problem. Blood flow to the injured area increases, arteries begin to dilate, and capillaries become more permeable so that white blood cells, hormones and other nutrients can flood into the injured tissue. White blood cells immediately begin ingesting germs, dead and damaged cells, and other foreign bodies in the affected area to support healing. Hormones called prostaglandins create blood clots to heal the damaged tissue and remove them when the tissue has healed.

This rush of blood to the injured area brings with it fluids that cause swelling, redness and heat that can trigger pain and fever. Pain is caused by the increased pressure that affects nerve endings. Pus can form if there is an excess of dead white blood cells. Superficial pus can be expelled through wounds in the skin surface, but puss that is embedded deeply in the body can only be extracted by inserting a needle into the area and drawing it out into a syringe, or in extreme cases, through surgery.

Inflammation is vital to healing because without it injuries and wounds would fester and the infections could eventually become septic. Untreated sepsis is a life-threatening condition. Pain and swelling also serve as an indicator that the body is in trouble and forces a slow-down, resulting in the necessary attention and rest the body needs to heal.

Bursitis pain can either be acute or chronic depending on its duration. Acute bursitis pain usually comes on suddenly and is sharp in quality. Acute pain usually does not last longer than six months and it goes away when the underlying bursitis condition has been alleviated. Chronic pain is pain that is ongoing and usually lasts longer than six months. This type of pain can continue even after the injury or illness that caused it has healed. Pain signals remain active in the nervous system for weeks, months, or years. Common symptoms of bursitis include:

- Pain in the region of the affected bursa
- Pain that is radiated or referred to other locations
- Tenderness over the affected bursa
- Limitation of movement over a joint surface
- Localized warmth over the surface of the affected bursa
- Localized redness over the surface of the affected bursa
- Pain around a joint surface that becomes worse during and after activity

1.2 Knee Bursitis Specifics

Knee bursitis is an inflammation of any of the bursae located within the knee joint. Knee bursitis is characterized by topical, localized swelling in the affected joint. It is a very painful condition that can dramatically affect knee mobility and execution of daily activities.

It is important to correctly diagnose the cause of knee pain to prevent the development of chronic inflammation that can persist for months and even years. Persistent chronic inflammation has been linked to heart disease, lung disease, kidney disease, cancer, degenerative bone disease, depression and more. The theory is that chronic inflammation does not lead to other diseases, but the presence of chronic inflammation combined with the potential for other disease encourages the development of other diseases.

Persistent knee pain that interferes with daily life must be addressed. A health care professional can diagnose knee bursitis by taking x-rays and possibly taking a sample of synovial fluid from the knee for analysis, if necessary. Synovial fluid is drawn from bursae with a needle and syringe in a process called arthrocentesis. It is a simple procedure where the joint area is first deadened with local anaesthetic, and after that a needle is inserted into the space between the bones of the joint to collect synovial fluid.

Knee bursitis is most commonly misdiagnosed as knee gout or knee tendonitis. Listed below are differences in symptoms of knee gout, knee tendonitis and knee bursitis.

Main symptoms of knee gout:

- Rapid onset of pain in the knee joint
- Warmth around the knee joint
- Swelling of the knee joint
- Reddish discolouration around the knee joint
- Limitation of motion

Main symptoms of knee tendonitis:

- A weakness of the knee
- Pain around the kneecap
- Pain when the kneecap is touched
- Pain after performing exercises that involve the knee joint

Main symptoms of knee bursitis:

- Pain around the knee joint
- Pain when pressure is applied to the knee joint
- Swelling of the knee joint
- A crepitating or "cracking" sound can be heard around the knee joint
- Pain can be sharp or dull depending on the amount of pressure within the knee bursa

1.3 Knee Bursae types

To obtain a clear and broad understanding of the condition, we would firstly need to be aware of the various bursae types present around the knee joint. These bursae are divided into three important groups, namely:

- *Frontal group*

The frontal group of bursae are located in front of the knee joint.

- *Medial group*

The medial group of bursae are located on the inner side of the knee joint.

- *Lateral group*

The lateral group of bursae are located on the outer side of the knee joint.

These groups consist of individual bursae that can exhibit inflammation in the occurrence of knee bursitis, and they are presented below:

Frontal group

- *Suprapatellar bursa*

The suprapatellar bursa is located between the frontal surface of the femur (the thigh bone) and the deep surface of a muscle known as the quadricep femoris.

- *Prepatellar bursa*

Prepatellar bursa is a bursa located in front of the patella (knee cap) bone.

- *Pretibial bursa*

The pretibial bursa is located between a part of the tibial bone (known as the tibial tuberosity) and the skin over that bone.

- *Subcutaneous bursa*

The subcutaneous bursa is located between subcutaneous tissues and sheets of fibrous tissues.

- *Deep infrapatellar bursa*

The deep infrapatellar bursa is a type of bursa found below the tendon of the kneecap (known as the patella tendon).

Medial group

- *Medial gastrocnemius bursa*

The medial gastrocnemius bursa is located between the inner head of the gastrocnemius muscle (known as the medial head) and the capsule of the knee joint.

- *Anserine bursa*

The anserine bursa is located between the ligament and tendons of the following muscles: sartorius, gracilis, and semitendinosus.

- *Bursa semimembranosa*

This bursa is located between the ligament and tendon of the semimembranosus muscle.

Lateral group

- *Fibular Bursa*

This bursa is located between the collateral ligament of the fibular bone of the leg and the tendons of a muscle known as biceps femoris.

- *Fibulopopliteal Bursa*

This bursa is located between the collateral ligament of the fibular bone of the leg and the tendons of a muscle known as popliteus.

- *Lateral Gastrocnemius Bursa*

The lateral gastrocnemius bursa is located between the outer head of the gastrocnemius muscle (known as the lateral head) and the capsule of the knee joint.

- *Subpopliteal Bursa*

This is a bursa located between the tendon of the popliteus muscle and the outer part of the femur bone, known as the lateral condyle of the femur.

1.4 Primary Knee Bursitis types

Knee bursitis can affect any of the bursae surrounding the knee joint, and the cause of the inflammation of any knee bursa can vary greatly. Anything from the natural ageing process, through to lifestyle and underlying disease can cause knee bursae to become inflamed, and sometimes the cause is unknown. Any type of knee bursitis can develop quite suddenly, or gradually over a period depending on the underlying cause. In the same way, any type of knee bursitis can last for few days, or persist for months, again depending on the underlying cause.

Any of the knee bursae that have been described so far can become inflamed or infected resulting in knee bursitis, but the most common types of knee bursitis (which are discussed in detail in later Chapters of this book) are the following:

- *Prepatellar Knee Bursitis*

Prepatellar knee bursitis is a painful condition in which there is swelling of the knee due to an inflammation of the prepatellar bursa. The prepatellar bursa is a small, balloon-like structure which is located in a soft tissue in front of the patella. The patella is a round, small bone located in the knee joint that is responsible for the extension movement of the knee. The main function of the prepatellar bursa is to reduce friction by acting as a separating medium between the patella and the patella tendons.

Bursitis of the prepatellar bursa is sometimes called carpet layer's knee, housemaid's knee or roofer's knee. It can be caused by a direct blow to the knee or from being in a prolonged kneeling position.

- *Pes Anserine Bursitis*

Pes anserine bursitis is an inflammation of the bursa located between the shinbone (tibia) and the three tendons of the hamstring muscle at the inside of the knee. It occurs when this bursa becomes irritated and produces too much fluid, which causes it to swell and put pressure on the adjacent parts of the knee.

The pes anserine bursa is a small, jelly-like sac that is located in the knee. Its location between the medial knee tendons and the tibia bone gives it a foot-like shape. The main function of the pes anserine bursa is to reduce friction by acting as a separating medium between the tibia bone and the hamstring muscle tendons.

Pes anserine bursitis is also known by other names such as Anserine Bursitis or Pes Anserinus Bursitis.

- *Infrapatellar Bursitis*

Infrapatellar bursitis is a painful inflammation of the infrapatellar bursa that can affect anyone, not just athletes or people with highly active lifestyles. The infrapatellar bursa is located beneath the knee cap, and it has two parts. The superficial infrapatellar bursa is found on top of the patellar tendon, while the deep infrapatellar bursa is found below the patellar tendon. Though there is an anatomic distinction between the two, clinically it is hard to tell the difference.

Infrapatellar bursitis is also known as 'clergyman's knee'. This is because the condition commonly occurs to people who kneel often.

- *Suprapatellar Bursitis*

Suprapatellar Bursitis is a pathological condition involving the knee in which there is inflammation of the suprapatellar bursa. 'Suprapatellar' simply means above the patella. Therefore, suprapatellar bursitis is the inflammation or swelling of the bursa located above the patella bone. Suprapatellar bursitis is very common in individuals who stress their knees by carrying heavy loads on a regular basis.

The exact location of the suprapatellar bursa is above the patella and between the distal femur (leg bone) and the quadriceps tendon. It permits free movement of the quadriceps tendon over the distal femur. It allows for full flexion (bending) and extension (straightening) of the knee. It can be irritated by a direct blow or from repeated stress or motions.

1.5 Septic Knee Bursitis

Septic bursitis occurs when any bursa becomes infected and is a potentially serious medical condition, particularly if left untreated. About 20% of all bursitis cases will become septic, and superficial bursae like those in the elbows, knees and shoulders, are more prone to becoming septic than bursae that are deeply embedded in the body. Septic bursitis always requires medical intervention because if left untreated, the infection can pass from the infected bursa into other parts of the body or the bloodstream.

There are factors that can increase the risk of septic knee bursitis. These include:

- An impaired response to infection due to an existing chronic medical condition
- Cancer
- Lupus
- Skin disease
- Kidney disease

- Steroid therapy
- Alcohol abuse
- Rheumatoid arthritis
- Type 1 or type 2 diabetes mellitus
- Chronic obstructive pulmonary disease
- Repeated bouts of non-infectious knee bursitis
- An open wound in the area of the knee bursae

All bursae risk becoming infected if they are punctured due to injury or medical procedures, and knee bursae are no exception. A puncture to a bursa can allow for bacteria or microorganisms to get inside and proliferate. Bursae can also become infected without any entry point in the skin, if there is an existing infection in the area of the joint, and in some cases the source of the infection is unknown. The assumption would be that bacteria are introduced into the bursa by infected blood passing through the joint.

If a knee bursa becomes infected, it will cause an inflammatory reaction in the body. The knee bursa will fill up synovial fluid, white blood cells and other components causing swelling, inflammation and pain. The mobility of the knee joint will become increasingly difficult. In addition to the symptoms experienced in the affected joint area, the patient will also begin suffering from a fever and chills and will start feeling gradually more ill. Septic bursitis causes the area to become red and hot to the touch.

If septic knee bursitis is suspected, antibiotic treatment will be started immediately, even before test results are available. Septic knee bursitis is almost always initially treated with intravenous antibiotics followed by a course of oral antibiotics. The earlier treatment begins, the less risk there is of complications. An antibiotic course should be between 10 to 14 days, with the bursal fluid being extracted at about three-day intervals for analysis, while antibiotics are being administered. Antibiotic treatment should be continued for at least five days after bursal fluid tests clear of infection.

Some doctors might opt for an ultrasound to detect the accumulation of bursal fluid, depending on the patient's circumstances. Infected synovial fluid could be drained from the infected knee bursa with a needle and syringe to lessen pressure and reduce infection. An infected knee bursa might need to be drained a few times to rid it totally of all the infected synovial fluid. If this is unsuccessful in curbing the infection, surgery might be required to drain the infected synovial fluid and treat the infection from inside the soft tissue of the knee joint.

With swift medical intervention and the right antibiotic treatment, septic knee bursitis should respond well to treatment. In rare cases, the infected knee bursa might be removed completely through surgery, particularly if there are recurrent bouts of septic or aseptic bursitis in the same knee bursa.

1.6 Knee Bursitis Facts and Statistics

Knee pain is one of the most common pains suffered by people in the United States of America as well as in the rest of the Western World. Knee bursitis is a very common cause of knee pain that can reoccur after healing depending on the cause. Knee bursitis is said to occur at least once in the lifetime of two in every one thousand people in the Western World.

Is Knee Bursitis Selective?

Knee bursitis is not a selective medical condition with regards to age or gender. Although knee bursitis shows more prevalence in women over the age of 40, no one is exempt. Knee bursitis can occur in children through to the elderly of both genders.

People over 40 years of age are more inclined to develop knee bursitis as a result of lifestyle or pre-existing health conditions, while people under the age of 40 are more inclined to develop knee bursitis as a result of injury or overuse of the knee joint due to excessive exercises, such as sport or dancing. Sickness at any age that results in extended bed rest or long periods of immobility can also trigger knee bursitis.

Knee bursitis does, however, show geographical selectivity, but there have not been many studies conducted on the geographical prevalence of the condition to date. From data available, there is definitely a higher prevalence of knee bursitis in Western World countries. The connection does not appear to be related to life expectancy, but rather to lifestyle. People from Western World countries are more inclined to adopt a sedentary lifestyle and consume a rich and unhealthy diet resulting in weight gain than people from the rest of the world. Also, people from Western World countries are more likely to partake in competitive activities where the desire to win or achieve a high level of skill and proficiency makes them push their bodies beyond healthy limits. In comparison, people from the rest of the world are more inclined to keep fit through doing daily chores well into old age for two reasons, namely:

- A culture that embraces everyone in the family as an active participating family member
- Economic factors that keep people working, including physical labor, to survive

By remaining physically active at a normal rate and avoiding excessive weight gain, people outside of the Western World countries and culture appear to be substantially less likely to develop knee pain and conditions like knee bursitis.

Effects of Weight and Lifestyle

Apart from injury or underlying disease, the most common causes of knee bursitis are related to diet and lifestyle. Knee bursitis that is not caused by disease or injury is caused by prolonged pressure on the knees or overuse of the knee joints. There are certain professions that cause daily pressure and strain on the knee joints as well as recreational activities that do the same. On the other hand, leading a sedentary lifestyle and gaining weight also puts strain and pressure on the knee joints.

Weight Gain and Leg Joints

Gaining too much weight can have a serious impact on your health and cause heart disease, high blood pressure, sleep apnea and Type 2 diabetes. But carrying too much weight also has a negative impact on bones, joints and muscles, and although the effects might not be potentially fatal, they can cause extreme pain, discomfort and impeded mobility.

Joints are designed to carry weight and cope with the stress of constant movement, but the design is intended to cope comfortably with a healthy weight only. The greater the body weight, the more stress is placed on joints, and the ankle joints, hip joints and knee joints in particular carry the brunt of the load. Although joint disease is not limited to people who are overweight, treating joint disease in overweight people is much more difficult than in people who are not overweight.

Clinical studies have confirmed that every extra pound or kilogram of weight a person carries exerts four times the amount of pressure on the ankle, hip and knee joints – so one extra pound exerts four pounds of pressure on the leg joints, or one extra kilogram exerts four kilograms of pressure on the leg joints. For example, a person who is ten pounds or kilograms overweight is exerting forty pounds or kilograms over and above the normal pressure on their leg joints every day with each step. Under these conditions bone, ligaments, muscle and tendons take massive strain as does everything surrounding the ankle, hip and knee joints, including bursae. This added daily strain eventually leads to inflammation in the area of the ankle, hip or knee joint, causing a wide range of complications including ankle bursitis, hip bursitis or knee bursitis. Ankle bursitis, hip bursitis or knee bursitis that is directly linked to excess weight can be very difficult to treat and can keep reoccurring unless the person loses the excess weight. Ankle bursitis, hip bursitis and knee bursitis that are caused by excess weight can severely affect a person's mobility, particularly if the condition keeps reoccurring and develops into a chronic condition.

Two other complications of carrying excess weight that can be directly linked to developing ankle bursitis, hip bursitis and knee bursitis are the following:

Firstly, people who are overweight are more likely to fall and injure themselves. This increases the chances of developing bursitis in any joint, but particularly in the hip joints and knee joints, because these joints usually take the most impact in a fall. If the skin around any bursae is broken during a fall, that can increase the chances of septic bursitis, because it will allow bacteria to enter the skin.

Secondly, people who are overweight are more inclined to dislocated joints, particularly dislocation of the hip joints and knee joints. Also, people who are overweight are inclined to arthritis, because the added pressure on joints causes the smooth joint surfaces to wear away. Both dislocation and arthritis can cause bursae in the affected joint to become inflamed, adding to the pain and discomfort of the underlying problem.

Effects of Lifestyle on Knee Joints

Knee bursitis is most often caused by repetitive motions, impact and overuse of a knee joint, or a direct minor impact on the outside of a knee joint. Knee bursitis can also be caused by a serious injury such as a motor vehicle accident or some similar knee trauma, but such cases are less common. Knee bursitis can be regarded as a common, everyday health condition.

Bad posture is also a very common cause of knee bursitis, and professions that involve repetitive joint motions can also be a cause. Sport, recreational activities, housework, gardening, handyman chores around the house – anything that involves repetitive motion of the knee joints - can spark off inflammation and result in knee bursitis. Daily activities that can cause knee bursitis include:

- Bending and lifting objects
- Carpentry
- Cycling
- Dancing
- Digging and shovelling
- Gardening
- Gymnastics
- Jogging and running
- Kneeling for prolonged periods of time
- Painting
- Scrubbing
- Sport (baseball, cricket, golf, tennis, etc.)

Any repeated activity that causes the contact oscillation of a knee joint, and/or constant impact with the ground can cause knee bursae to become irritated and inflamed resulting in knee bursitis. Also, a minor fall or bump against a knee joint can potentially lead to irritation and swelling resulting in knee bursitis.

Symptoms of knee bursitis can develop very suddenly leaving the patient immobile and in severe pain. In healthy people, knee bursitis should begin to heal within a few days after resting the joint and using methods to relieve the pain. It can, however, reoccur if the person resumes the activity that caused the condition. If that happens, it will require a rethink of how daily activities are conducted. A physical therapist will be able to assist with exercises to strengthen muscles and connective tissue around the knee joint, but if the condition persists a visit to a physician is best.

Effect of existing medical conditions

Neurological conditions
Apart from underlying medical conditions that can make a person more susceptible to knee bursitis, there are certain neurological conditions that predispose people to injury that can cause trauma to knee joints.

These include epilepsy, seizure disorder, ataxia (a lack of voluntary coordination of muscle movements), dementia and organic disease.

Rheumatoid arthritis and gout

Rheumatoid arthritis affects the synovial membranes surrounding joints, including the knee joints, and people who suffer from rheumatoid arthritis of the knee are more likely to get knee bursitis because of the existing inflammation in the knee joints. Although gout in the knee joints is not so common, people who do suffer from gout in the knee joints are also more likely to develop knee bursitis. Gout is a painful inflammatory condition caused by a build-up of urate crystals in the synovial joints.

Musculoskeletal disorders

Existing physical conditions that alter the musculoskeletal functions of the lower limbs can have a knock-on effect that results in knee pain. For instance, arthritis and osteoarthritis have been associated with an increased risk of developing knee bursitis. Also, people who have one leg longer than the other, even by a small margin, may adopt a gait that irritates the knee bursa leading to knee bursitis. Another trigger that can increase the risk of developing knee bursitis is knee surgery or surgery near the knee joint.

Immune system suppression

Certain medical conditions greatly suppress the immune system or create a need for people to be treated with medications that suppress the immune system. Lifestyle choices can also suppress the immune system. A suppressed immune system makes a person more susceptible to developing septic bursitis, including septic knee bursitis. Health conditions or lifestyle choices that can suppress the immune system include:

- Autoimmune disease (diabetes, lupus, rheumatoid arthritis, etc.)
- Certain types of cancer
- Chemotherapy
- Radiation therapy
- Chronic Obstructive Pulmonary Disease (COPD)
- Drugs prescribed after organ transplants
- Human Immunodeficiency Virus (HIV) that causes *Acquired Immune Deficiency Syndrome* (AIDS)
- Alcoholism
- Drug addiction
- Obesity

- Severe stress

Bone spurs or calcium deposits

Soft tissue in a knee joint, including knee bursae, can become irritated by bone spurs or calcium deposits known as osteophytes. Osteophytes in the knee form when a knee joint has been affected by arthritis. Osteoarthritis damages cartilage and this results in bone rubbing on bone. The damaged bones compensate for the loss of cartilage by growing outwardly and forming soft calcium deposits that harden into bone spurs. Osteoarthritis develops slowly and the pain and inflammation it causes worsens over time, potentially leading to further complications in the knee joint, like knee bursitis.

Chapter 2: Prepatellar knee bursitis

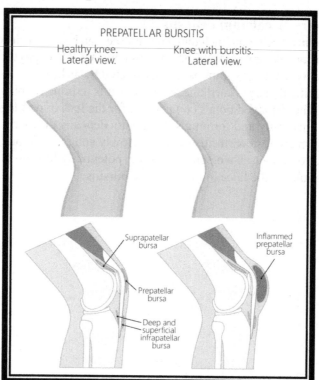

As the name of this condition would suggest, prepatellar knee bursitis is characterized by inflammation of the prepatellar bursa located in a soft tissue in front of the patella

Prepatellar bursitis is also known by several other names such as beat knee, carpet layer's knee, coal miner's knee and housemaid's knee.

In this chapter, you will learn all there is to know about prepatellar knee bursitis including the bursa anatomy and the condition causes, signs, symptoms, diagnosis, complications and prognosis.

2.1 Anatomy of the Prepatellar Bursa

The prepatellar bursa is a small, balloon-like structure that is located in a soft tissue in front of the patella. The patella is a round, small bone located in the knee joint, which is responsible for the extension movement of the knee. That is where this bursa derives its name from; "pre-patellar" means before the patella.

The main function of the prepatellar bursa is to reduce friction by acting as a separating medium between the patella and the patella tendons.

2.2 What Causes Prepatellar knee bursitis?

Prepatellar bursitis is usually caused by a repeated, excessive pressure on the knees. This is why the condition is common among people whose job requires them to kneel constantly. Typical examples of these occupations are carpet layers, coal miners, roofers, plumbers and housemaids.

In addition, studies have shown that the following factors are likely to cause prepatellar knee bursitis:

- Obesity: Being obese or overweight puts a lot of pressure on the knee joint and could put you at a risk of prepatellar bursitis.
- Arthritis: Arthritis (which is a disorder of the joint) can also cause prepatellar knee bursitis.
- Trauma to the knee: It could be in the form of a fall or a blow to the knee.
- Gout: Crystals from gout may be deposited in the knee joint and it may predispose you to the condition.
- Sarcoidosis: This is a disease that causes deposition of inflammatory cells in some parts of the body. Deposition of some of these cells in the knee could cause prepatellar bursitis.
- Diabetes mellitus: It has been reported in the medical literature that diabetes mellitus increases the risk of prepatellar knee bursitis.
- Alcohol overconsumption can put you at risk of developing prepatellar knee bursitis.
- Increased pressure on a previously injured knee during activities such as climbing the stairs, running or hiking.

2.3 Signs and Symptoms of Prepatellar Bursitis

If you notice any of the following signs and symptoms, you should consider seeing a Doctor, because you may have prepatellar knee bursitis:

- Prominent swelling around the kneecap: This swelling is a result of the accumulation of fluid around the kneecap.
- Redness over the area of swelling: The skin above the prepatellar bursa appears very red.

- Decreased movement over the knee joint: The knee joint is unable to perform movements like flexion and extension due to the fluid that has accumulated around the knee joint and the pain felt when movement is attempted.
- Pain over the patella, when it is touched and when you want to rise from a sitting position.
- Crepitus of the knee joint: Crepitus is a cracking or creaking sound heard around the knee of people with prepatellar knee bursitis, when they attempt to make movement around the knee joint.
- Warmth of the swollen surface: When the swollen surface of the knee is touched, it feels warm.

2.4 Diagnosing Prepatellar Bursitis

Prepatellar bursitis can be accurately diagnosed by a qualified medical professional. The doctor will first ask you a few questions and then carry out an examination of the affected region.

Medical History

The information given to the doctor will help in the diagnosis of prepatellar bursitis. Here are some questions you may be asked:

- Knee pain: When did the knee pain start? What time of the day does the knee hurt you the most? How severe is the knee pain?
- Swollen knee: When did the knee swelling start?
- Difficulty while walking: How difficult has walking been since the knee swelling started?
- Inability to bend or kneel with the affected knee: How far can you bend the knee without it hurting you?
- Having a job or occupation that requires constant kneeling: How often do you kneel?
- History of trauma to the knee: Did you fall on your knee? Did anything hit your knee?

Physical Examination

After collecting the relevant information that will help diagnosis, the doctor will go ahead to examine you and take note of the following:

- Pain on the knee when it is touched
- Redness of the skin over the knee joint
- Reduced flexion of the knee

- Warmth over the surface of the knee (it can indicate that the knee is infected)

Aspiration of the content of the bursa

This means that a needle is used to take out some of the fluid from a swollen bursa and this fluid is examined in the laboratory for the following:

- Urate crystals found in gout
- Pyrophosphate crystals found in pseudo-gout
- An evidence of an infective process going on such as an increase in the number of white blood cells
- Cholesterol crystals, which are usually found in rheumatoid bursitis.

Imaging tests

Imaging tests are tests performed to view certain parts of the body that cannot be seen from outside using special machines.

For prepatellar knee bursitis, the common imaging tests employed are:

- Plain X-ray
- Magnetic Resonance Imaging (MRI)
- Computed Tomography Scan (CT)
- Ultrasound

2.5 What Are the Treatment Options?

If you are able to avoid the activity that caused your prepatellar knee bursitis in the first place for an extended period of time, it may heal on its own. Unfortunately, this would mean severely limiting your mobility and that might not be an option for you. Your other options include medical treatments to reduce inflammation and relieve pain as well as physical therapy or assistive devices. Please refer to subsequent chapters for generic knee bursitis treatment options.

The most common medications used to treat prepatellar knee bursitis include non-steroidal anti-inflammatory drugs (NSAIDs), such as ibuprofen and naproxen. These drugs will help reduce the inflammation in your knee joint and, hopefully, in doing so, relieve some of the pain. Unfortunately, these drugs have a risk of side effects such as stomach pain or bleeding, so it is recommended that you only take them for a short period of time.

Another option for the treatment of prepatellar knee bursitis is steroid injections. These injections allow your doctor to deliver corticosteroid medication directly into the joint to reduce swelling and relieve pain. This therapy often works well in conjunction with physical therapy exercises aimed at improving and maintaining strength and flexibility in the knee joint. You might also use an assistive device such as a cane, walker, or crutches to take the weight off your knee as it heals.

In cases where none of the treatment mentioned above are sufficient to relieve your pain, surgery is an option. It is possible to remove the affected bursa through a laparoscopic procedure – this is when a surgeon makes a small incision and performs the surgery using camera guidance. In most cases, the recovery period is just a few days.

2.6 Tips to Prevent Prepatellar Knee Bursitis

In most cases, prepatellar knee bursitis is caused by overuse. That means that the best way to prevent the problem is to avoid the activities that cause it. Unfortunately, you probably can't avoid walking or climbing stairs, but there are certain precautions you can take when exercising or performing these activities:

- Go slow – if you're just starting an exercise program, take it easy and slowly build up the intensity.
- Limit yourself – when exercising, keep the weight low and limit the number of repetitions.
- Keep an eye on your pain – it is normal to feel a little bit of discomfort when you are working hard, but stop if it becomes unusually painful.

It is also a good idea to lose weight if you're overweight or obese, because that extra weight is putting additional strain on your knees and other joints. Avoid repetitive activities that strain the knees and make sure you wear supportive, properly fitted shoes. If you need additional support, walk with a cane or crutches.

In addition to taking these general precautions, Chapter 6 presents some exercises you can do to maintain the strength and flexibility of your knee and surrounding muscles in order to prevent and treat prepatellar knee bursitis.

2.7 Complications and Prognosis

Without treatment, prepatellar knee bursitis has the potential to worsen over time and the pain may eventually come to impact your daily activities. If the condition worsens, you may lose range of motion in your knee and could even develop a physical disability. Fortunately, non-invasive treatments such as exercise, physical therapy, and medications are successful in relieving prepatellar knee bursitis in as many as 90% of cases. There are even exercises you can do and precautions you can take to prevent the problem from recurring.

Chapter 3: Pes Anserine Knee Bursitis

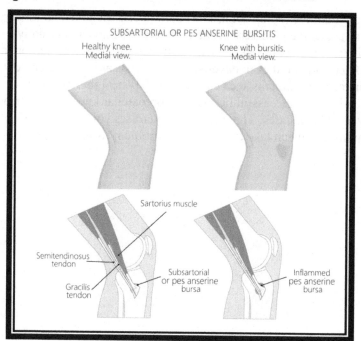

Pes anserine bursitis is an inflammation of the bursa located between the shinbone (tibia) and the three tendons of the hamstring muscle at the inside of the knee. It occurs when this bursa becomes irritated and produces too much fluid, which causes it to swell and put pressure on the adjacent parts of the knee.

Pes anserine bursitis is also known by other names such as Anserine Bursitis or Pes Anserinus Bursitis.

3.1 Anatomy of the Pes Anserine Bursa

The pes anserine bursa is a small, jelly-like sac that is located between the medial knee tendons and the tibia bone of the knee. Pes anserine means *"goose's foot"* in Latin.

This bursa has a foot-like shape and its main function is to reduce friction by acting as a separating medium between the medial knee tendons and the tibia bone of the knee joint.

3.2 What Causes Pes Anserine Bursitis?

Pes Anserine bursitis is usually caused by repetitive activities (like squatting, stair climbing, etc.) which result in tightness of the hamstring muscles. This tightness places more pressure on the pes anserine bursa and causes an irritation of the bursa, which eventually results in the inflammation or swelling of the bursa.

Other common causes of pes anserine bursitis include the following:

- Obesity: Being obese or overweight is a risk factor for pes anserine bursitis
- A degenerative joint disease which specifically affects the knee, such as arthritis
- Flat feet: Which is also known as pes planus, can put you at risk of pes anserine bursitis
- Sporting activities that require a lot of sideways movement, such as tennis
- The tightness of the tendons in the knee joint
- Trauma to the knee: It could be a fall or a blow to the knee
- Diabetes mellitus: Studies have shown that diabetes mellitus contributes significantly to the risk of having pes anserine bursitis
- Increased pressure on a previously injured knee

3.3 Signs and Symptoms of Pes Anserine Bursitis

As is true for all forms of bursitis, the primary symptom associated with pes anserine bursitis is pain. Pain related to pes anserine bursitis is typically experienced at the kneecap when it is touched and when you want to rise from a sitting position. Pain can also come on slowly after a vigorous and long training session.

Because pes anserine bursitis can sometimes be confused with other conditions, your doctor will need to perform some tests in addition to a physical exam and a review of your symptoms. Here are some of the signs your doctor may look for to diagnose pes anserine bursitis:

- Prominent swelling around the kneecap: This swelling is as a result of the accumulation of fluid around the kneecap.
- Redness over the area of swelling: The skin above the pes anserine bursa appears very red.

- Decreased movement over the knee joint: The knee joint is unable to perform movements like flexion and extension, due to the fluid that has accumulated around the knee joint and the pain felt when movement is attempted.
- Crepitus of the knee joint: Crepitus is a kind of creaking sound heard around the knee of people with pes anserine knee bursitis when they attempt to make a movement around the knee joint.
- Warmth around the swollen surface: When the swollen surface of the knee is touched, it feels warm to touch.

If left untreated, these symptoms may worsen over the course of weeks or months. As the pain worsens, it may lead to limping. If you experience this kind of pain, it is a good idea to talk to your doctor to get a proper diagnosis.

3.4 Diagnosing Pes Anserine Bursitis

Pes Anserine bursitis can be accurately diagnosed by a qualified medical doctor. The professional will ask you a few questions and carry out an examination of the affected region.

Medical History

The information given to the Doctor will help in the diagnosis of pes anserine bursitis. Here are some questions you may be asked:

- Knee pain: When did the knee pain start? What time of the day does the knee hurt you the most? How severe is the knee pain?
- Swollen knee: When did the knee swelling start?
- Difficulty while walking: How difficult has walking been since the knee swelling started?
- Inability to bend or kneel with the affected knee: How far can you bend the knee without it hurting you?
- Job or occupation that requires constant kneeling: Does your job require you to kneel frequently?
- Trauma to the knee: Did you fall on your knee? Did you hit your knee on anything?
- Tight hamstring muscles: How tight are your hamstring muscles? Are your hamstrings usually sore?
- Pain while standing after being in a seated position: Do you usually feel pain in your knee region when you are about to stand up?

- Muscle overuse from athletic activities: The doctor will ask if you are an athlete or if you are constantly involved in sporting activities.
- Medical records of previous degenerative disease of the knee: The doctor will ask if you have previously had any degenerative disease in your knee, such as arthritis.

Physical Examination

After collecting the relevant information that will help diagnosis, the doctor will now go ahead to examine you and take note of the following:

- Pain on the knee when it is touched: The pain of pes anserine bursitis is usually mild to moderate. An increased intense pain could point to other medical conditions, like a fracture
- Palpation of the hamstring muscles will show a significant amount of tightness
- Redness of the skin over the knee joint
- Reduced flexion of the knee
- Inability to extend your knee in chronic cases of pes anserine bursitis
- Warmth over the surface of the knee can indicate that the knee is infected

Aspiration of the content of the bursa

This means that a needle is used to take out some of the fluid from a swollen knee and this fluid is examined in the laboratory for the following:

- Urate crystals
- Pyrophosphate crystals
- An evidence of an infective process going on such as an increase in the number of white blood cells
- Your current cholesterol crystals
- Gram staining: This is a test done to examine fluid gotten from the body for the presence of bacteria

Imaging tests

Common imaging tests performed in cases of pes anserine bursitis are the following:

- Plain X-ray to check if the bone is affected
- Magnetic Resonance Imaging (MRI)
- Computed Tomography Scan (CT)
- Ultrasound: To check for the amount of fluid deposited around the soft tissues in the knee joint.

Based on the results of these tests, your doctor will be able to tell you if you have pes anserine bursitis and, from there, you'll be able to discuss your treatment options and make the best choice.

3.5 What Are the Treatment Options?

The treatment for pes anserine bursitis will vary depending on the underlying cause as well as the severity of the condition. In mild cases of pes anserine bursitis, resting the joints and using home remedies to reduce inflammation and relieve pain may be adequate. For example, applying a cold compress or ice pack to the affected joint may help with the pain (see subsequent Chapters for more home remedies that could provide relief). Modifying your daily activity or exercise routine to avoid repetitive motions may help as well.

In more severe cases of pes anserine bursitis, you may need to use a cane or crutches to relieve some of the pressure on the joint and ease the pain. Medical treatments like over-the-counter anti-inflammatories, such as acetaminophen, aspirin, and ibuprofen, may help to reduce inflammation and relieve pain as well. If those don't work, talk to your doctor about a corticosteroid injection directly into the bursa. Physical therapy may also help to stretch the knee and strengthen the knee muscles. Also, refer to subsequent chapters for generic knee bursitis treatment options.

3.6 How to Prevent Pes Anserine Bursitis

In most cases, pes anserine bursitis is caused by repetitive activities and overuse. That means that the best way to prevent the problem is to avoid the activities that cause it. Unfortunately, you probably can't avoid walking or climbing stairs, but there are certain precautions you can take when exercising or performing these activities:

- Wear kneepads often
- Avoid direct trauma to your knee
- Rest your knees regularly after a period of intense use
- Apply ice to your knees after a period of intense use

3.7 Complications and Prognosis

Because the symptoms of pes anserine bursitis are likely to worsen over time, it is important to get them checked out by your doctor. If left untreated, the pain can get much worse. There is also the risk that the bursa could rupture and become infected. Infections like this are rare, but the signs may include:

- Fever or chills
- Worsening joint pain
- Warm, inflamed skin
- Feeling sick

With proper treatment, the prognosis for pes anserine bursitis is very good. In many cases, modifying your activity and taking pain medications will help to reduce inflammation and relieve pain. During treatment you should avoid activities that put repetitive stress on the knees.

Chapter 4: Infrapatellar Knee Bursitis

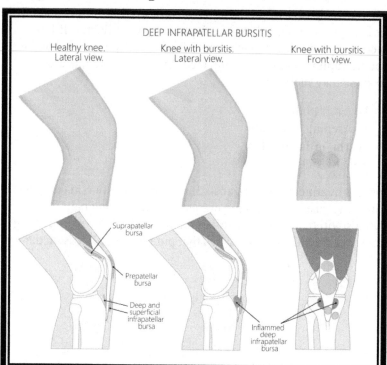

Infrapatellar bursitis occurs when one or both of the infrapatellar bursae sacs inside the knee become irritated and inflamed resulting in swelling and knee pain. 'Infrapatellar' simply means below the patella. Therefore, infrapatellar bursitis is the inflammation or swelling of the bursae located below the patella bone.

Infrapatellar bursitis is also known as 'clergyman's knee'. This is because the condition commonly occurs to people who kneel often.

4.1 Anatomy of the Infrapatellar Bursa

The infrapatellar bursa is a small jelly-like sac which contains fluid and is located in the knee below the kneecap (patella). The fluid it contains is known as synovial fluid and it is rich in protein and collagen. These fluid-filled sacs are located in areas where two surfaces in your body (most often where a bone and tendon or a bone and muscle) rub together during movement.

There are two infrapatellar bursae within the knee, namely:

- The superficial infrapatellar bursa: This bursa is located between a connective tissue (known as the patella tendon) and the skin. It acts as a sort of cushion between these two structures.
- The deep infrapatellar bursa: This bursa lies below the kneecap between the patella tendon and the upper front surface of the tibia (shin bone).

Though there is an anatomic distinction between the two, clinically it is hard to tell the difference on which one is inflamed.

4.2 What Causes Infrapatellar Bursitis?

Infrapatellar bursitis is usually caused by the overuse of the infrapatellar bursae. Also, any form of excessive force on or a breakdown of the tissue which protects the kneecap can result in a case of infrapatellar bursitis.

Other common causes of infrapatellar bursitis include:

- Obesity: Being obese or overweight means that your knee has to carry more weight and this can result in the irritation of the bursae of the knee. Such irritation can lead to infrapatellar bursitis.
- Trauma: Application of excessive pressure to the knee at the top of the shin bone can cause injury to the infrapatellar bursa (for example, a fall).
- Pressure: Excessive stress on the knee joint can lead to infrapatellar knee bursitis.
- Other diseases of the joint: A degenerative joint disease which specifically affects the knee, such as arthritis. can cause infrapatellar bursitis.
- Knee overuse: Athletes who overuse their knees despite an injury to the knee can be at risk of developing the condition.
- Infection: Since the superficial infrapatellar bursa is close to the surface of the knee, an untreated cut on the surface of the knee near the bursa can put you at risk of developing septic infrapatellar bursitis.

4.3 Signs and Symptoms of Infrapatellar Bursitis

If you notice any of the following signs and symptoms, then you should consider seeing a doctor, because you may have infrapatellar knee bursitis:

- Pain over the patella when it is touched and when you want to rise from a sitting position.
- Prominent swelling around the kneecap: This swelling is due to the accumulation of fluid around the kneecap.
- Redness over the area of swelling: The skin above the infrapatellar bursa appears very red.
- Limited range of motion of the knee joint: The knee joint is unable to perform movements like flexion and extension due to the fluid that has accumulated around the knee joint and the pain felt when movement is attempted.
- Difficulties Sleeping: Patients suffering from infrapatellar knee bursitis may have interrupted sleep patterns. Simply bending the knee or rolling over during sleep can cause pressure on the inflamed bursa, increasing the pain. The pain can range from mild to very sharp depending on the amount of swelling and inflammation of the bursa. Placing a pillow between your knees/thighs while you sleep might help reduce pain throughout the night.
- Crepitus of the knee joint: Crepitus is a cracking or creaking sound heard around the knee of people with infrapatellar knee bursitis. when they attempt to make movement around the knee joint.
- Warmth of the swollen surface: When the swollen surface of the knee is touched, it feels warm to touch.

4.4 Diagnosing Infrapatellar Bursitis

When you are experiencing knee pain, a visit to the doctor is always recommended, as there are many conditions that can cause knee pain such as a meniscus tear, an ACL sprain, patellar or quadriceps tendinitis, a fracture, and also infrapateller knee bursitis. Getting a proper diagnosis is important so you can treat your condition correctly.

To start with, your doctor will gather a medical history about you, your current condition and your symptoms. He/she will ask about the amount and nature of pain you are having at your knee. How long you have had your symptoms and if you have range-of-motion loss with your leg and knee. Details about what caused the pain in the knee, when it started, and whether or not you have ever had treatments for this or a similar condition in the past are also very helpful in assessing your injury.

A physical examination will subsequently be performed to determine if you have any signs of infrapatellar knee bursitis or other knee injury. The medical professional will visually assess and palpate (feel) the bones and soft tissue in both your knees to evaluate any differences between the two of them. This will identify any abnormalities, such as swelling, bone deformities, atrophied muscles, redness and/or warmth on the skin. In many cases, the first sign that you have infrapatellar knee bursitis is swelling around the kneecap.

If a soft tissue injury is suspected, an MRI may be performed to view where and how extensive the damage is. An x-ray might be recommended to rule out a bone spur or other foreign body as the cause of your knee pain.

As the superficial infrapatellar bursa is close to the surface of the skin, it is more susceptible to septic, or infectious, bursitis caused by a cut or scrape on the knee. Septic bursitis requires antibiotics to get rid of the infection. Your doctor will be able to determine whether there is an infection or not by drawing a small sample of the bursa fluid with a needle.

4.5 How to Prevent Infrapatellar Bursitis

Some simple recommendations that can help you prevent infrapatellar knee bursitis, especially if the sport you participate in puts you at risk of the disease:

- Wear kneepads often
- Avoid direct injury to your knee
- Rest your knees regularly after a period of intense use
- Apply ice to your knees after a period of intense use

4.6 Complications

Because the symptoms of infrapatellar knee bursitis are likely to worsen over time, it is important to get them checked out by your doctor. If left untreated, the pain can get much worse. There is also the risk that the bursa could rupture and become infected. Infections like this are rare, but they are still a possibility.

With proper treatment, the prognosis for infrapatellar knee bursitis is very good. In many cases, modifying your activity and taking pain medications will help to reduce inflammation and relieve pain. During treatment you should avoid activities that put repetitive stress on the knees.

Chapter 5: Suprapatellar Knee Bursitis

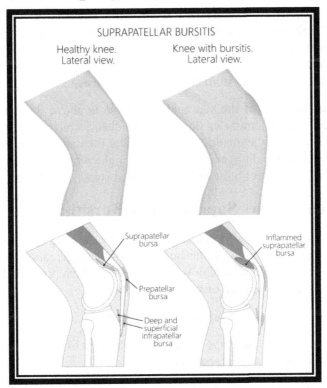

Suprapatellar knee bursitis is the last knee bursitis type we will be discussing in this book before we look in detail how you can treat knee bursitis in the next chapter.

Suprapatellar bursitis is a pathological condition involving the knee in which there is inflammation of the suprapatellar bursa. 'Suprapatellar' simply means above the patella. Therefore, suprapatellar bursitis is the inflammation or swelling of the bursa located above the patella bone. Suprapatellar bursitis is very common in individuals who stress their knees by carrying heavy loads on a regular basis.

The suprapatellar bursa is vulnerable to injury from both acute trauma and repeated microtrauma. Acute injuries might be from direct trauma to the bursa via falls directly onto the knee, as well as from overuse injuries, including running on soft or uneven surfaces, or from jobs that require crawling on the knees, such as carpet laying.

5.1 Anatomy of the Suprapatellar Bursa

The suprapatellar bursa is a small, balloon-like structure which contains synovial fluid and is located in the knee above the kneecap. The knee joint is made up of certain bones and ligaments. Bursae, such as the suprapatellar, are crucial for a normal knee joint function, because they prevent these structures from constantly rubbing against one another.

The exact location of the suprapatellar bursa is above the patella and between the distal femur (leg bone) and the quadriceps tendon. It permits free movement of the quadriceps tendon over the distal femur. It allows for full flexion (bending) and extension (straightening) of the knee. It can be irritated by a direct blow or from repeated stress or motions.

5.2 What Causes Suprapatellar Bursitis?

Suprapatellar knee bursitis is usually caused by the excessive and frequent use of the suprapatellar bursae. Also, the application of an excessive force on or a breakdown of the tissue which protects the patella can result in a case of suprapatellar bursitis.

Other common causes of suprapatellar bursitis are the following:

Repetitive Stress: Excessive stress on the knee by lifting heavy objects repetitively can cause suprapatellar knee bursitis.

Trauma: Application of enormous pressure to the knee at the top of the femur bone can cause injury to the suprapatellar bursa, for example, a fall or vehicle collision. Excessive stress on the knee joint can lead to suprapatellar bursitis.

Other diseases of the joints: A degenerative joint disease which specifically affects the knee, such as arthritis, can pose you at risk of developing suprapatellar knee bursitis.

Knee overuse: Athletes who overuse their knees despite a previous injury can develop suprapatellar knee bursitis.

Gout: This condition causes the deposition of crystals in certain joints of the body. Deposition of gout crystals in the knee joint can put your knees at risk of developing suprapatellar bursitis.

Lupus Erythematous: This is an inflammatory disease in which the immune system of the body attacks certain body tissues. People with lupus have also been noted to develop suprapatellar bursitis.

Note: The suprapatellar bursa is close to the surface of the knee. Thus, an untreated cut on the skin near the bursa can put you at risk of developing septic suprapatellar bursitis.

5.3 Signs and Symptoms of Suprapatellar Bursitis

If you notice any of the following signs and symptoms, then you should consider consulting a doctor because you may be suffering from suprapatellar bursitis:

- Dull, achy pain or tenderness above the knee joint
- Prominent swelling around the kneecap
- Redness over the swollen area
- Limited movement range of the knee joint: The knee joint is unable to perform movements like flexion and extension due to the fluid that has accumulated around the knee joint and the pain felt when movement is attempted.
- Crepitus of the knee joint: Crepitus is a cracking or creaking sound heard around the knee of people with suprapatellar knee bursitis when they attempt to make movement around the knee joint.
- A feeling of warmth on the swollen surface: When the swollen surface of the knee is touched, it feels warm to touch.

You might feel these symptoms when you put pressure on the area through activities such as kneeling, jumping, or running. You may also feel symptoms when you are resting. Also, depending on what caused your bursitis, symptoms may come on suddenly or gradually. For instance, symptoms may come on suddenly if you were to take a hard fall onto your knee. Conversely, symptoms may appear more slowly when there is repeated use or stress to the area, such as from kneeling often or for extended periods.

5.4 Diagnosing Suprapatellar Bursitis

Suprapatellar bursitis can be accurately diagnosed by a qualified doctor. The professional will ask you a few questions and carry out an examination of the affected region.

Medical History

The history you will be providing will help in the diagnosis of the condition. Some of the questions you will be asked include:

- Knee pain: When did the knee pain start? What time of the day does the knee hurt you the most? How severe is the pain?
- Swollen knee: When did the knee swelling start?
- Difficulty while walking: How difficult has walking been since the knee swelling started?
- Inability to bend or kneel with the affected knee: How far can you bend the knee without it hurting you?
- Having a job or occupation that requires constant kneeling: Does your job require you to kneel frequently?
- History of trauma to the knee: Did you fall on your knee? Did anything hit your knee? Were you involved in an accident?
- History of previous knee bursitis: Have you had knee bursitis before? How long did it last? How did you treat it?

Physical Examination

After collecting the medical history, the doctor will go ahead to examine you and take note of the following:

- Pain intensity and location on the knee when it is touched.
- Redness of the skin over the knee joint.
- Reduction in the flexion movement of the knee.
- Reduction in the extension movement of the knee.
- Warmth over the surface of the knee.
- An increased body temperature could indicate that you might have septic knee bursitis, which requires urgent treatment.

Aspiration of the Suprapatellar Bursa

This means that a needle is used to take out some of the fluid from the bursa and this fluid is examined in the laboratory for the following:

- Urate crystals
- Pyrophosphate crystals
- An evidence of an infective process going on, such as an increase in the number of white blood cells
- Cholesterol crystals
- Gram staining

Imaging tests

Imaging tests are largely done to show or to know what is going on in the body that is not visible to the naked eyes.

Some common imaging tests required to diagnose suprapatellar bursitis are:

- X-rays: These are usually taken to check if the bones are also involved in the condition.
- Magnetic Resonance Imaging (MRI): Performed to locate the exact bursa that is inflamed.
- Ultrasound: May help in the application of injection to the bursa or help during aspiration of the bursa.

5.5 How to Prevent Suprapatellar Bursitis

Some simple recommendations that can help you prevent suprapatellar knee bursitis, especially if the sport you participate in or the daily activity you indulge in puts you at risk of the disease, are the following:

- Wear kneepads often: Wearing kneepads reduces the risk of irritation to the knee bursae, hence reducing the risk of suprapatellar bursitis.
- Avoid direct injury to your knee.
- Rest your knees regularly after a period of intense use.
- Apply ice to your knees after a period of intense use.

5.6 What are the treatment options?

The treatment options for suprapatellar knee bursitis can include the following:

- resting and avoiding activities that could irritate the area, such as kneeling, jumping, or running
- taking over-the-counter pain medication such as Ibuprofen (Motrin, Advil) and acetaminophen (Tylenol) to help relieve pain and swelling
- applying an ice pack in the area to ease swelling (remember to never apply an ice pack directly to your skin, but wrap it in a towel or cloth first
- using a knee brace to stabilize and limit movement of the knee
- taking a course of antibiotics if an infection is present (take the entire course, even if you begin to feel better)

If your bursitis is not responding to standard treatment, your doctor may choose to inject a corticosteroid into the affected area to relieve swelling in the absence of infection.

In some cases, your doctor may recommend physical therapy to help with strength and flexibility in the area surrounding your knees. This can help reduce stress on the knee and may also reduce the risk of a recurrence.

Severe or recurring cases of suprapatellar bursitis may also be treated through drainage or surgical removal of the suprapatellar bursa.

Please refer to subsequent Chapters for a more detailed discussion on the various treatment options

5.7 Prognosis

With proper treatment, the prognosis for suprapatellar bursitis is very good. In many cases, modifying your activity and taking pain medications will help to reduce inflammation and relieve pain. During treatment you should avoid activities that put repetitive stress on the knees.

Chapter 6: Knee Bursitis Treatment

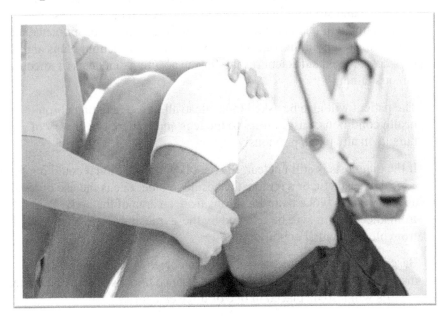

Knee bursitis treatment is mostly by oral medicines, topical medicines, physical therapy and rest. Invasive treatment through fluid drainage or surgery is uncommon except in the case of septic knee bursitis.

6.1 Knee Bursitis Diagnosis

Knee pain is a very common symptom of numerous conditions of the legs, making a diagnosis of any condition very complex. An external examination is not likely to be sufficient to diagnose knee bursitis. Some of the bursae in the knees are deeply embedded in the soft tissue around the knee joints, and there are few if any external symptoms of knee bursitis present. Diagnosis of knee bursitis relies on an accurate clinical assessment, so a consultation with a healthcare professional will include a thorough analysis of the patient's lifestyle and each symptom to identify or exclude any other conditions that might be present. The patient will also be taken through a series of physical knee joint resistance and rotational tests and the extraction of bursal fluid for analysis might be necessary. A Magnetic Resonance Imaging (MRI) scan, ultrasound or X-rays are also alternative options a healthcare professional has at their disposal. These will identify any calcification present around a knee bursa or enlargement of a knee bursa.

The standard process of diagnosis will follow the set approach of physical inspection of the patient's knee, the range of motion, stability, resistance and strength in the affected knee. Based on this assessment, the decision will be made whether bursal fluid needs to be extracted and if a scan is required. In some cases, bursal fluid extraction, scans and X-rays do not yield sufficient results for the accurate diagnosis of knee bursitis either.

The patient will also be asked to disclose all past or existing chronic health conditions, past injuries to the legs and if there is a history of bursitis in any joints previously.

If the diagnosis is still unclear, the healthcare professional could opt for a local anaesthetic or a regional anaesthetic bloc; this is the use of local anaesthetics to block pain sensations from an area of the body. Pain from knee bursitis will be relieved by these injections, and so identify it from other potential conditions.

Based on these assessments and their outcomes, a diagnosis will be made to confirm and identify the type of knee bursitis present. The knee bursitis will also be placed in one of three categories:

- Acute knee bursitis: that occurs as a result of trauma to the knee joint, or massive overload.
- Chronic knee bursitis: that occurs as a result of overuse or excessive pressure on the knee joint. Muscle strain can also be a cause.
- Septic knee bursitis: that occurs when bacteria have infiltrated the knee bursa and the synovial fluid has become infected.

6.2 Clinical Treatment of knee Bursitis

Once there is a firm diagnosis, and the type of knee bursitis has been identified, treatment can commence. Treatment depends on the level of severity of the knee bursitis more than it depends on the type of knee bursitis diagnosed. Treatment includes immediate measures to address the condition and can also include recommendations to make certain lifestyle changes.

There are several different treatments for aseptic knee bursitis, and patients can be treated with any one or combination of these treatments based on the diagnosis and the patient's immediate circumstances. Treatment for knee bursitis is mostly home treatment with visits to relevant healthcare professionals to monitor the healing progress and administer additional treatment. It is seldom that a patient will be hospitalized to treat knee bursitis on its own. If there is a different underlying condition that is causing the knee bursitis, that condition could require hospitalization to treat it effectively.

Septic knee bursitis is the exception and is always regarded as a medical emergency. On diagnosis, it is treated with an intravenous antibiotic immediately, and hospitalization might be required depending on the patient's condition and circumstances. If the intravenous treatment yields positive results, treatment can be continued at home with a course of oral antibiotics that will be combined with treatments similar to those for aseptic knee bursitis.

Assistive walking devices, such as a walking stick or crutches, might be prescribed for a few days or a few weeks to aid mobility while the knee bursae are healing. Orthopaedic pads or cushions might be prescribed to allow for comfortable sitting and lying down.

Pain relief is always the first step in treating any type of knee bursitis, because knee pain is the most prominent symptom and it is the main reason most patients seek medical help. After that, management of pain in the affected knee, as the inflamed bursae take time to heal, is the next step.

6.3 Pain Relief

- Steroid injections: They are often used to treat knee bursitis, because the bursae are deeply embedded in the soft tissue around the knee. Usually, a corticosteroid together with a local anaesthetic are injected directly into the affected knee bursa immediately after diagnosis. Often, only one injection is needed to bring relief and facilitate the healing process of the knee bursa. If pain and inflammation reoccur in the same knee bursa, another injection can be administered, and even a third injection can follow, but each injection must be separated by a few weeks at least. Patients must rest the knee for at least three days after each injection for maximum effect. Prolonged use of corticosteroid can potentially damage the soft tissue surrounding the knee bursae and knee joint leading to further medical complications.
- Oral drugs: Prescriptions of oral non-steroidal anti-inflammatory drugs are the most common form of pain relief treatment for knee bursitis. Non-prescription over-the-counter

anti-inflammatory drugs are also effective to relieve and control pain.

- Topical anti-inflammatory treatments: Gels and balms can be helpful if the affected knee area allows for pressure and massage. These treatments offer relief once the healing has already begun and the swelling has started to subside, and the knee joint is more mobile.
- Ice pack: Ice packs effectively reduce swelling and ease the pain. Because certain knee bursae are deeply embedded in the soft tissue of the knee joint, ice is not effective in treating all types of knee bursitis. Treatment with ice packs will mostly be done during physical therapy sessions.
- Warm compress: a warm compress increases blood circulation and raises the skin temperature. A warm compress can be a better option to soothe painful muscles and pain located deep in the knee area. Treatment with a warm compress will mostly be done during physical therapy sessions.

6.4 Surgery

Surgery is always a last resort, even in cases of septic knee bursitis, and is recommended in instances where all other attempts of treatment have been unsuccessful and all options have been exhausted. Surgery is recommended to treat and drain the infected synovial fluid in septic knee bursitis or to remove thickened knee bursae and any bone spurs that are present in the case of aseptic knee bursitis. Sometimes affected tendons are treated at the same time. Rarely, afflicted knee bursae are surgically removed to address recurring problems. This procedure is known as a bursectomy.

6.5 Physical Therapy

Physical therapy will be prescribed to treat knee bursitis, depending on the degree of severity and the patient's circumstances. In some cases, physical therapy will only commence once there are signs of healing, particularly in the case of septic knee bursitis. The recommended exercises can be done at home or under the care of a professional physical therapist.

In the first few weeks, physical therapy will focus on heat treatments and passive stretching exercises to reduce pressure and pain. As the knee bursa begins to heal, the focus will shift to improving flexibility, muscle strength and joint mobility. Physical therapists might also use electrotherapy, acupuncture and soft tissue massage to relieve pain and get rid of stiffness in the surrounding muscles.

Physical therapy follows a program, starting with pain and stress relief and then moving on to strengthening and stretching muscles and introducing exercises that will allow the patient to resume their normal activities without relapse. Depending on the severity of the knee bursitis and the patient's circumstances, physical therapy can be recommended for a few days, weeks or months. The healing process will set the pace and time necessary. Further details on physical therapy are discussed in later Chapter on alternative pain treatment.

6.6 Exercises that Alleviate Symptoms

It is very important to note that physical exercise must only be done if knee bursitis has been diagnosed by a healthcare professional, who has recommended physical exercises to promote healing. Self-diagnosis is not recommended, and physical exercise can do more harm than good, if the underlying cause of knee pain has been misdiagnosed. Also, in the instance of septic knee bursitis that has not been diagnosed and treated by a healthcare professional, physical exercise will not aide the infected knee bursa in any way, but could cause further irritation and the spread of inflammation.

In the case of medical conditions of the knee like knee bursitis, rest is usually more beneficial in the early stages of healing, and the pain cannot be exercised away. Once healing has begun, a regular exercise program will strengthen weakened muscles. The success of rehabilitation through exercise will depend on the patient's commitment to follow an exercise program.

An otherwise healthy patient should exercise twice a day, every day to aid recovery from knee bursitis. Each exercise should be repeated ten times in the first week after recovery, fifteen times in the second week and twenty times after the third week. If exercising at home, find a comfortable place with plenty of space to exercise. A bed with a firm mattress makes an excellent place to exercise safely and comfortably if the exercise requires you to be lying down.

Physical exercise must always be conservative, if knee bursitis has been diagnosed, unless the patient is under the direct care and instruction of a physical therapist. Otherwise, keep the exercise routine simple and manageable.

The following 17 exercises are uncomplicated, can easily be done at home, and can benefit healing from knee bursitis:

1. **Hamstring stretch on wall**

    Lie on your back with the buttocks close to a doorway. Stretch your uninjured leg straight out in front of you on the floor through the doorway. Raise your injured leg and rest it against the wall next to the door frame. Keep your leg as straight as possible. You should feel a stretch in the back of your thigh. Hold this position for 15 to 30 seconds. Repeat 3 times.

2. **Standing calf stretch**

    Stand facing a wall with your hands on the wall at about eye level. Keep the injured leg back with your heel on the floor. Keep the other leg forward with the knee bent. Turn your back foot slightly inward (as if you were pigeon-toed). Slowly lean into the wall until you feel a stretch in the back of your calf. Hold the stretch for 15 to 30 seconds. Return to the starting position. Repeat 3 times. Do this exercise several times each day.

3. **Quadriceps stretch**

    Stand at an arm's length away from a wall with your injured side furthest from the wall. Facing straight ahead, brace yourself by keeping one hand against the wall. With your other hand, grasp the ankle on your injured side and pull your heel toward your buttocks. Don't arch or twist your back. Keep your knees together. Hold this stretch for 15 to 30 seconds.

4. **Quad sets**

    Sit on the floor with the injured leg straight and your other leg bent. Press the back of the knee of your injured leg against the floor by tightening the muscles on the top of your thigh. Hold this position 10 seconds. Relax. Do 2 sets of 15.

5. **Heel slide**

    Sit on a firm surface with the legs straight in front of you. Slowly slide the heel of the foot on your injured side toward your buttock by pulling your knee toward your chest as you slide the heel. Return to the starting position. Do 2 sets of 15.

6. Straight leg raise

Lie on your back with the legs straight out in front of you. Bend the knee on your uninjured side and place the foot flat on the floor. Tighten the thigh muscle on your injured side and lift your leg about 8 inches (20 centimetres) off the floor. Keep your leg straight and your thigh muscle tight. Slowly lower your leg back down to the floor. Do 2 sets of 15.

7. Side-lying leg lift

Lie on your uninjured side. Tighten the front thigh muscles on your injured leg and lift that leg 8 to 10 inches (20 to 25 centimeters) away from your other leg. Keep the leg straight and lower it slowly. Do 2 sets of 15.

8. Wall squat with a ball

Stand with your back, shoulders, and head against a wall. Look straight ahead. Keep the shoulders relaxed and your feet 3 feet (90 centimeters) from the wall and shoulder's width apart. Place a soccer or basketball-sized ball behind your back. Keeping your back against the wall, slowly squat down to a 45-degree angle. Your thighs will not yet be parallel to the floor. Hold this position for 10 seconds and then slowly slide back up the wall. Repeat 10 times. Build up to 2 sets of 15.

9. Quadriceps isometrics

Sitting on the floor with your injured leg straight and your other leg bent, press the back of your knee into the floor by tightening the muscles at the top of your thigh. Hold this position for 10 seconds. Relax. Do 3 sets of 10.

10. Hamstring isometrics

Sitting on the floor with your injured leg slightly bent, dig the heel of your injured leg into the floor and tighten up the back of your thigh muscles. Hold this position for 5 seconds. Do 3 sets of 10.

11. Long Arcs

Sit on the edge of a chair. Kick your leg out straight. Hold for about 2 seconds. Return your leg back to the initial resting position and repeat several times.

12. Hamstring isometrics

Lie flat on your back with your leg straight out. Place an object known as a bolster under the affected knee. Slowly straighten your knee until your leg is fully straight with the bolster beneath your knee. Tighten your quadriceps muscles. Do 3 sets of 10.

13. Hip and knee reflex

Lying on the back with both legs straight, and working each leg separately, gently bend the hip and knee joints by sliding the heel towards the buttock while keeping the heel on the exercise surface. Make sure to keep the kneecap pointing straight at the ceiling. Gently slide the heel back again, until the leg is straight. Repeat with the other leg. Keep each leg bent for five seconds before straightening it again. Relax and repeat the routine.

Note: it might be more comfortable to wear a pair of thin socks when doing this exercise, if it causes friction on the heels.

14. Standing Knee Stretch

Stand with one arm resting on a supportive surface. Pick up your foot at the ankle and bent it up toward your back. Hold this position for about 30 seconds, then switch to the other knee.

15. Partial Squat

Stand with feet about hip-width apart. Place your hands straight out in front of you for balance. Slowly sit back and bend at the knees until you are in a seated position. Hold for about 5 seconds, then slowly stand. Repeat this exercise 10 times.

16. Heel Raise

Stand with your hands on the back of a chair for support. Lift your uninjured knee off the ground. Stand on the toes of your other foot. Slowly raise and lower your heel 10 times. Switch to the other leg and repeat.

17. Leg Push

For this exercise, you will need a resistance band. Lie on your back with your legs stretched out straight. Lift one foot with your knee at a 90-degree angle. Wrap a resistance band around your foot and hold the two ends in your hands. Push against the band with your leg while holding the ends in your hands. Hold for 2 seconds. Repeat 10 times, then switch to the other leg.

6.7 Exercises that Aggravate Symptoms

There are certain exercises that must definitely be avoided by patients recovering from knee bursitis. Because knee bursitis affects the muscles and nerves in the knee joint, care must be taken not to aggravate the condition during the healing process. Aggravating knee bursae during the healing process can cause knee bursitis to flare up again.

All exercises that place intense stress or impact on the knee joints must be avoided for at least one month after the knee bursitis has healed, because although the patient might be pain-free, there could still be mild inflammation in the knee joint. This is particularly true if a patient has been treated with pharmaceutical drugs to ease the pain. Strong drugs can mask pain, giving the patient a false sense of security.

The following four types of exercise must be avoided by patients recovering from knee bursitis:

1. **Cardiovascular Exercises**
   Although cardiovascular exercises are known to aid recovery from illness, they place significant stress and impact on the knee joints. Working out with cardio-equipment, jogging, running, cycling, aerobics, etc. must be avoided until all inflammation in the knee joint has healed.
2. **Contact Sports**
   Knee joints play a major role in all contact sports and are therefore very vulnerable to injury. Impact, pivoting and twisting can take their toll on inflamed knee joints. Sports like basketball, golf, soccer (football) and tennis must be avoided until all inflammation in the knee joint has healed.
3. **Strengthening Exercises**
   Strengthening exercises place significant stress and impact on the knee joints. They also involve sequences of repetitive joint movements that include the knee joints. This includes using

exercise machines that require bending the knees or shaking the legs. Although some of these exercise machines may not be designed to work the knees, the movements can take their toll on inflamed knee joints. Lunges, deep squats and any other repetitive movement that places severe stress on the legs and knees must be avoided until all inflammation in the knee joint has healed.

Other exercises that exert too much pressure on the knee joint and should be avoided during the knee bursitis rehabilitation period include the following:

- Hurdler's stretches
- Jumping rope
- Deep lunges
- Single leg squat
- Duck walks
- Plyometric exercises
- Straight leg sit-ups
- Standing straight leg toe touch

Chapter 7: Pharmaceutical Medication

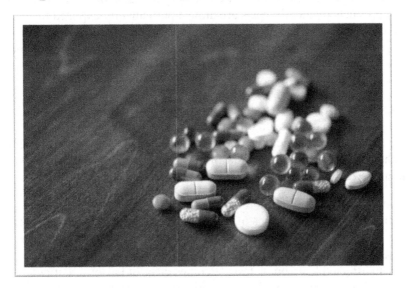

Pharmaceutical drugs are used to diagnose, cure, treat or prevent disease. Drug therapy relies on the science of pharmacology for continual advancement. Pharmaceutical drugs are manufactured by strict chemical processes, even if the key components of a drug are derived from a natural source.

7.1 Antibiotics

Antibiotics are a type of drug used to treat and prevent bacterial infection in the human body. Depending on the type and purpose of an antibiotic, they can either kill or inhibit the growth of bacteria. Antibiotics are only effective for the treatment of bacterial infections; they are not effective for treating viral infections.

Because of the overuse of antibiotics over the past century, many strains of bacteria have developed a resistance to treatment. Drug-resistant bacteria is such an extreme problem worldwide that the World Health Organization has classified it as a serious threat that has the potential to affect anyone of any age in any country. The overuse of antibiotics does not only lie in over-prescription, but also in the widespread and ever-increasing use of antibiotics in commercial farming. Commercial farmers constantly feed livestock and poultry antibiotics, as a prophylactic to prevent sickness rather than to treat sickness. A sick animal or bird costs money to treat, and it might die before it has yielded any profit. People who consume meat, poultry and dairy products on a daily basis are almost permanently exposed to antibiotics, so when they contract an infection, the antibiotics prescribed have little effect. Buying certified organic meat, poultry and dairy products ensures that the products are free of antibiotics among many other harmful components.

Antibiotics are only used to treat septic knee bursitis. The infected synovial fluid that has been drawn from an infected knee bursa is analyzed to make an accurate diagnosis and identify the type of bacteria that has caused the infection. Antibiotics will be prescribed and administered based on the analysis results.

In most patients, the infection clears completely after two weeks of antibiotic treatment. In cases of severe infection, the infection can take up to four weeks to clear. Healthcare professionals will recommend a further five-day course of oral antibiotics after the synovial fluid drawn from an affected knee bursa tests becomes clear of bacteria. Patients who suffered severe septic knee bursitis or recurring bouts of knee bursitis should have follow-up tests for up to six months to ensure that the synovial fluid in the affected knee bursa remains bacteria free.

Bacterial infections in knee bursae are most commonly caused by staphylococcus and streptococcus bacteria. Antibiotics usually prescribed to clear these bacterial infections are dicloxacillin, oxacillin, and penicillin. These antibiotics are packaged and sold under different brand names. Penicillin is the most widely used antibiotic against infections caused by staphylococci and streptococci bacteria, but many bacteria have developed a resistance to it because of overuse. Dicloxacillin is mostly prescribed in instances of penicillin resistance.

Side Effects

About 1 in 15 people will experience side effects when taking antibiotics, because antibiotics affect people differently. Some people experience no side effects at all, while other people can experience side effects ranging from mild to severe. In most cases, a patient can persevere through mild side effects, because the benefit of the antibiotic outweighs the negative impact of the side effects. In more severe cases, the antibiotic use must be stopped immediately because the side effects can have a dire effect on the patient's health and can in some cases be fatal.

Any side effects must be reported to the health professional who prescribed the antibiotic, even if they are mild. In some cases, the side effects might be because the dose is too high. In those instances, reducing the dosage will eliminate the side effects and the patient can still benefit from the antibiotic treatment.

Common side effects of antibiotics include:

- Nausea
- Diarrhea
- Vomiting
- Stomach cramps
- Thrush: oral and vaginal (yeast infections)
- Swollen tongue
- Persistent headache

Serious side effects of antibiotics include:

- Fever, chills and body aches
- Any flu-like symptoms
- Sore throat
- Uncharacteristic weakness
- Bloody diarrhea
- Dark urine
- Urinating less than usual or not urinating at all
- Yellowing of the skin or whites of the eye
- Skin rash, blistering or peeling
- Bruising easily or bleeding under the skin
- Agitation or confusion
- Seizures

Allergy

About 10% of patients report an allergic reaction to antibiotics, in particular, penicillin. However, serious allergic reaction occurs in only 0.03% of these patients. An allergic reaction can occur within minutes of taking antibiotics, or within a few hours. In some cases, an allergic reaction can occur after a day or two as levels of the antibiotic build up in the body. Any allergic reaction to antibiotics must be reported to a healthcare professional immediately. Allergic reactions are known as anaphylaxis and can rapidly become fatal with patients dying within minutes.

Symptoms of an allergic reaction include:

- Flushing of the skin
- A sense of panic
- Hives (bumps) all over the body or in patches
- Red and itchy eyes
- Swelling of the face, mouth and throat
- Difficulty speaking and swallowing
- Shortness of breath, wheezing and coughing
- Severe asthma
- Sudden drop in blood pressure
- Collapse and unconsciousness
- Seizures
- Low platelet or red blood cell count

7.2 Non-Steroidal Anti-Inflammatory Drugs

Prescription and over-the-counter drugs are the first line of defence for treating aseptic knee bursitis. Non-steroidal anti-inflammatory drugs work by blocking the enzyme cyclooxygenase that produces prostaglandins. Although there are many contributors to the inflammatory process, prostaglandins play a significant role in the spread of inflammation. They cause increased blood flow, chemotaxis (chemicals that trigger an immune response), and add to dysfunction of tissue and organs. Without cyclooxygenase, there is no prostaglandin production and therefore no pain, fever, swelling and inflammation.

Over-the-counter anti-inflammatory drugs containing aspirin, naproxen and ibuprofen are the most widely prescribed and recommended. These drugs treat a broad range of medical conditions including pain, fever, and strained and sprained muscles. Their effect is short-term and treats the symptoms of a condition and not the cause. They can also be used for post-surgery pain relief.

Corticosteroids are another type of non-steroidal anti-inflammatory drug. They reduce inflammation and swelling by reducing the production of a range chemicals involved in inflammation. They reduce the activity of white cells as well, and this can have a negative impact on the immune system if they are used over an extended period.

Non-steroidal anti-inflammatory drugs are very effective in treating inflammatory conditions (such as knee bursitis), and there are unfortunately few other options available to patients. Patients who experience side effects, allergy or are considered too high risk to use non-steroidal anti-inflammatory drugs on a regular basis can discuss very low doses combined with alternative treatments with a healthcare professional.

Side Effects

Unfortunately, not everyone can use non-steroidal anti-inflammatory drugs, particularly if there is another underlying health condition that will be aggravated by the treatment. The most common existing conditions negatively affected by non-steroidal anti-inflammatory drugs are heart disease and inflammatory diseases of the gastrointestinal tract, like stomach ulcers. People who have these conditions are considered high risk for developing complications.

In some instances, high-risk patients can safely take low doses of non-steroidal anti-inflammatory drugs under the supervision of a healthcare professional. In these cases, long-term use should be avoided, because the longer a patient is exposed to the harmful compound in the drugs the more likely they are to develop side effects. Also, there are people who develop allergic reactions to non-steroidal anti-inflammatory drugs. This is referred to as sensitivity or intolerance rather than an allergy on package inserts.

Side effects for high-risk patients using non-steroidal anti-inflammatory drugs include:

- Increased risk of heart attack. This particularly affects men over 40 years of age who are overweight, smoke, have high blood pressure, high cholesterol and have previously suffered a stroke or heart attack.
- Increased risk of internal bleeding and reduced clotting of blood.

Although there are no completely safe non-steroidal anti-inflammatory drugs, it is suggested that naproxen may be less risky. Tramadol is also considered less risky, but it has a high potential for dependence which must be considered and weighed up against the benefits.

Allergy

Allergic reactions to non-steroidal anti-inflammatory drugs are quite common. While some sources rate it higher, the accepted percentage of people who report allergies is about 20% of patients treated. Any allergic reaction to non-steroidal anti-inflammatory drugs must be reported to a healthcare professional immediately. Allergic reactions are known as anaphylaxis and can rapidly become fatal with patients dying within minutes. An allergic reaction can occur within minutes of taking the drugs, or within a few hours. In some cases, an allergic reaction can occur after a day or two as levels of the non-steroidal anti-inflammatory drugs build up in the body.

Symptoms of an allergic reaction include:

- Flushing of the skin
- A sense of panic
- Hives (bumps) all over the body or in patches
- Red and itchy eyes
- Swelling of the face, mouth and throat
- Difficulty speaking and swallowing
- Shortness of breath, wheezing and coughing
- Severe asthma
- Sudden drop in blood pressure
- Collapse and unconsciousness
- Seizures
- Low platelet or red blood cell count

Patients who suffer from asthma, nasal polyps, chronic sinusitis or chronic hives are more inclined to develop an allergic reaction to non-steroidal anti-inflammatory drugs. This allergic reaction can inflame and worsen the existing condition.

7.3 Paracetamol (Acetaminophen)

Paracetamol (also known as acetaminophen) is sold worldwide under various brand names as over-the-counter and prescription drugs. It is available in tablet, capsule, syrup and powder format, and is often combined with other components to treat specific health conditions, like coughs and influenza. Paracetamol belongs to a class of drugs known as analgesics and antipyretics. Analgesics relieve pain, and antipyretics reduce fever. The mechanisms of paracetamol are not well understood, but it is believed that it reduces the production of prostaglandins in the brain, which results in curbing pain and fever. Prostaglandins are chemicals that cause swelling and inflammation in the body that leads to fever.

Paracetamol is very effective for treating mild to moderate pain in the body, including muscle and joint pain. It can be effective in treating knee bursitis, but it has a limited effect on treating inflammation. Using paracetamol in conjunction with other pain treatments will make it more effective. Paracetamol is an alternative for people who cannot use non-steroidal anti-inflammatory drugs because there are other underlying health conditions that will be aggravated by the treatment.

People who have a history of alcoholism or suffer from liver disease must not use any medication containing paracetamol, unless prescribed by a healthcare professional who is aware of their medical history. People who are taking chronic medication for unrelated health conditions must also first check with a healthcare professional before taking paracetamol.

Side Effects

Paracetamol is considered to be a reasonably safe drug, if taken in a daily dosage of 1000mg (usually two 500 mg tablets or capsules) four times a day with at least four hours separating each dose. No more than 4000mg of paracetamol is recommended in every 24-hour period. It is also recommended that paracetamol not be taken for more than ten days consecutively.

Most people tolerate paracetamol well, if used as recommended because it does not irritate the gastrointestinal system, like many other painkilling drugs do. Paracetamol does, however, carry a very strong caution of potential liver damage if the daily dose is exceeded, or if it is overused over an extended period.

Common side effects that range from minor to moderate include:

- Nausea and vomiting
- Loss of appetite
- Stomach pain
- Dry mouth, nasal passages and throat
- Blurred vision
- Dizziness
- Drowsiness

If these or any other symptoms occur and persist or worsen when taking paracetamol, stop using it immediately. If paracetamol has been prescribed by a healthcare professional, advise them as soon as possible.

Very serious side effects are seldom experienced but are definitely not improbable. Serious side effects include:

- Severe stomach pain accompanied by nausea, vomiting or diarrhoea
- Dizziness, sweating and fainting
- General weakness, shakiness and fatigue
- Unusual bruising
- Dark urine
- Urinating less than usual or not urinating at all
- Yellowing of the skin or whites of the eye
- Confusion or hallucinations

Any of these side effects must be reported to a healthcare professional immediately without delay.

Allergy

Allergic reactions to paracetamol are not very common. An allergic reaction can occur within minutes of taking paracetamol, or within a few hours.

Symptoms of an allergic reaction include:

- A rash breaking out anywhere on the body
- Red and itchy eyes
- Swelling of the face, mouth and throat
- Difficulty speaking and swallowing
- Shortness of breath, wheezing and coughing
- Sudden drop in blood pressure
- Collapse and unconsciousness
- Seizures

Any symptoms of potential allergy must not be ignored and must be reported to a healthcare professional immediately without delay. Although paracetamol is considered to be a reasonably safe drug, it is not necessarily compatible with everyone and consequences of allergy can in some cases be fatal.

Chapter 8: Alternative Pain Treatments

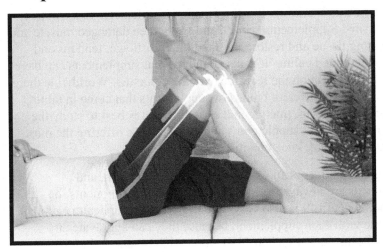

Pharmaceutical drugs are not the only way to control pain. There are many natural medicines and remedies that can be used to compliment pharmaceutical drugs when treating knee bursitis. Taking a holistic approach to treating knee bursitis can be very beneficial, because few medical conditions occur in isolation. For people who have allergies too or those who suffer from the side effects of pharmaceutical drugs, these options are a valuable course of action. In all cases, embracing alternative treatments will most likely do more good than harm. Even in cases of septic knee bursitis where antibiotic treatment is not negotiable, introducing alternative treatments will benefit the patient in the long term.

Alternative treatments include lifestyle changes, regular exercise, natural medicines, natural remedies and holistic medicine. If a patient is considered high risk because of any existing medical conditions, or if the patient is being treated for any other chronic medical conditions, the alternative treatments must be discussed with a healthcare professional to ensure that they do not impede existing treatment in any way.

One of the best alternative treatments for knee bursitis is rest. Even if a patient is undergoing physical therapy to facilitate healing and aid the strengthening of muscles and tendons, rest is still vital for recovery from all types of knee bursitis. Keep in mind that knees are weight-bearing joints, even when sitting, so they are easily stressed if they are injured, and inflammation can be easily aggravated.

8.1 Supplements

There are a number of off-the-shelf natural supplements that can treat knee bursitis. Supplements rebuild and strengthen damaged muscle and surrounding tissue and restore muscle tissue, cartilage, tendons and bone to facilitate healing. It is also believed that supplements can have a prophylactic effect on the recurrence of knee bursitis. Worldwide there are thousands of different brands of supplements that come in tablet, capsule, effervescent, tincture and syrup form. It is best to study the contents of different supplements and choose those offering the most benefits for treating knee bursitis.

No single component can work successfully on its own, and supplements are always made up of a number of components for maximum benefit. It is also very important to read the health cautions that come with each supplement, because they can aggravate any existing health issues such as high blood pressure and kidney disease.

The following supplements can treat knee bursitis:

- **Avocado Soybean Unsaponifiables (ASU):** ASU is natural vegetable extract made from one-third avocado oil and two-thirds soybean oil. ASU blocks pro-inflammatory chemicals, prevents deterioration of synovial cells which line the joints, and may help regenerate normal connective tissue. Clinical studies have shown that if ASU is taken regularly, it can reduce the need for nonsteroidal anti-inflammatory drugs. Available in soft gel capsules and oil, the recommended dosage is 300mg per day. Check the packaging to see how much needs to be taken daily to reach the recommended dosage.
- **Boron:** Boron is a trace mineral that is essential for the proper absorption and metabolism of calcium, copper and magnesium. Together these four trace minerals are vital to building proper bone health. Boron is present in a number of foods, and a healthy diet should provide enough to maintain bone health. Available in capsules and tablets, the recommended dosage is 3.25mg per day. Check the packaging to see how much needs to be taken daily to reach the recommended dosage.
- **Boswellia Serrata:** Boswellia serrata supplements are derived from the gum resin of the Boswellia trees found in India. It is commonly known as frankincense and is widely recognized for its powerful anti-inflammatory and pain relief properties. It also

improves joint mobility. Available in capsules and tablets, the recommended dosage is 450mg per day divided into three doses of 150mg each. Check the packaging to see how much needs to be taken daily to reach the recommended dosage.

- **Calcium: Calcium** is a mineral that occurs naturally in the human body that maintains strong bones and teeth, regulates muscle contractions, transmits nerve impulses, and helps release essential hormones and enzymes. Available in capsules, powder and tablets, the recommended dosage to treat conditions like knee bursitis is 1500mg (1.5g) per day divided into two doses of 750mg each. Once the knee bursitis has healed, a daily dose of 1000mg (1g) is recommended to maintain healthy joints. Check the packaging to see how much needs to be taken daily to reach the recommended dosage.

- **Cat's claw:** Cat's claw supplements are derived from the bark of a woody vine known as Uncaria Tomentosa that originates from South America. It has anti-inflammatory and analgesic properties, and clinical studies have found that it effectively reduces inflammation, pain and swelling in joints. Available in capsules, tablets and liquid, the recommended daily dosage is 350mg. Check the packaging to see how much needs to be taken daily to reach the recommended dosage.

- **Chondroitin sulfate:** Chondroitin is a natural substance found in the human body. It is a vital component of bone and cartilage, that helps draw water and nutrients into the cartilage to keep it healthy. Chondroitin sulfate supplements contain chondroitin that has been extracted from animals. Chondroitin sulfate supplements complement the existing chondroitin in the human body and aid to reduce pain and inflammation and improve joint function. It is also believed to enhance the effectiveness of collagen, block enzymes that break down cartilage, and help cartilage retain water. Available in capsules, tablets and powder, the recommended dosage is 800mg to 1200mg (1.2g) per day divided into four doses. Check the packaging to see how much needs to be taken daily to reach the recommended dosage.

- **Coenzyme Q10:** Coenzyme Q10 is a natural substance that occurs in the mitochondria of human cells and is vital to cell health. Clinical studies have shown that coenzyme Q10 can reduce inflammation and cell stress. When taken regularly, it can reduce degenerative cartilage breakdown. Coenzyme Q10 supplements are a yeast derivative and are mostly available in capsules. The recommended dosage is 90mg to 120mg per day. Check the packaging to see how much needs to be taken daily to reach the recommended dosage.

- **Curcuma longa:** Curcuma longa supplements are derived from the roots of the turmeric plant, that is commonly used as a spice in Asian cuisine. It has been used for centuries in Traditional Chinese Medicine and Indian Ayurvedic Medicine to treat inflammatory conditions amongst others. Clinical studies have shown that curcuma longa is very effective in reducing and preventing joint inflammation, pain and swelling. Available in capsules, extract and powder, the recommended dosage is 1g per day divided into two doses of 500mg each. Check the packaging to see how much needs to be taken daily to reach the recommended dosage.

- **Devil's claw:** Devils claw is a herb that originates from South Africa and has been used in local traditional medicine for centuries. It contains an active ingredient known as harpagoside, that is responsible for its anti-inflammatory and analgesic properties. Clinical studies have shown that devil's claw is effective in treating joint pain and improving joint mobility. Available in capsule, extract, powder and tincture, the recommended dosage is 2250mg (2.25g) per day divided into three doses of 750mg each. Check the packaging to see how much needs to be taken daily to reach the recommended dosage.

- **Gamma Linoleic Acid (GLA):** GLA is an Omega-6 fatty acid that is found in blackcurrant oil, borage oil and evening primrose oil. Clinical studies have shown that GLA is effective in treating joint pain, stiffness and swelling. Available in capsules and oil, the recommended daily dosage is 2000mg (2g) to 3000mg (3g) divided into two or three doses. Check the packaging to see how much needs to be taken daily to reach the recommended dosage.

- **Ginger:** Ginger supplements are derived from the roots of the ginger plant commonly used as a spice in Asian cuisine. It has been used for centuries in Traditional Chinese Medicine and Indian Ayurvedic Medicine to treat inflammatory conditions amongst others. Clinical studies have shown that ginger is as effective at reducing inflammatory reactions in cells as pharmaceutical steroids. Available in capsule, extract, powder and tincture, the recommended dosage is 3000mg (3g) per day divided in two to four doses. Check the packaging to see how much needs to be taken daily to reach the recommended dosage.

- **Glucosamine:** Glucosamine is a natural substance found in the human body, and it is a vital component of healthy joint cartilage. Glucosamine supplements are derived from shellfish and plant sources. Glucosamine supplements complement the existing glucosamine in the human body and help draw water and nutrients into cartilage to prevent degeneration. Clinical studies have shown that glucosamine is effective in reducing joint pain and stiffness, and also improves joint function. Available in capsules, tablets, liquid and powder, the recommended dosage is 1500mg (1.5g) per day divided into doses of 500mg each. Check the packaging to see how much needs to be taken daily to reach the recommended dosage.

- **Magnesium:** Magnesium is a mineral that occurs naturally in the human body and plays a crucial role in maintaining health. Magnesium is vital for healthy bones, muscles and nerves among many other important functions. Available in capsules and tablets, the recommended dosage is 1500mg (1.5g) per day divided into doses of 500mg each. Check the packaging to see how much needs to be taken daily to reach the recommended dosage.

- **Methylsulfonylmethane (MSM):** MSM is an organic sulphur compound that occurs naturally in the human body, where it aids in forming new and maintaining existing healthy connective tissue. Supplements are derived from animals, fruit and vegetables. MSM reduces joint pain and inflammation. Clinical studies have found that MSM is an effective natural analgesic and also improves joint mobility. Available in capsules, liquid, powder and tablets, the recommended dosage is 6000mg (6g) per day divided into three doses of 2000mg (2g) each. Check the packaging to see how much needs to be taken daily to reach the recommended dosage.

- **Omega-3 fatty acids:** There are two types of omega-3 fatty acids that are derived from fish oil, namely docosahexaenoic acid (DHA) and eicosapentaenoic acid (EPA). Clinical studies have shown that both DHA and EPA reduce pain, inflammation and swelling. Supplements are widely available, but many experts recommend that fresh fish is a preferred source of DHA and EPA. Available in gel capsules and oil, the recommended dosage is 3000mg (3g) per day. Check the packaging to see how much needs to be taken daily to reach the recommended dosage.

- **Propolis:** Propolis is produced by bees to maintain the sterility of beehives. Propolis supplements are made of pure propolis extracted directly from beehives. Apart from its antibacterial, antifungal and antimicrobial properties, clinical studies have shown that propolis also has anti-inflammatory and analgesic properties. Available in capsules, liquid and tincture, the recommended dosage is 500mg per day. Check the packaging to see how much needs to be taken daily to reach the recommended dosage.

- **Pycnogenol:** Pycnogenol is an extract from the maritime pine tree that originates from the Mediterranean. It contains an active ingredient known as *procyanidin,* that is a powerful anti-oxidant inhibiting pro-inflammatory enzymes. Clinical studies have shown that pycnogenol effectively reduces joint pain and stiffness and improves joint mobility. Available in capsules and tablets, the recommended dosage is 150mg per day. Check the packaging to see how much needs to be taken daily to reach the recommended dosage.

- **Vitamins:** Vitamins are essential to maintaining general health. Some vitamins build bone, cartilage and muscles, while others can protect against inflammation. Vitamins that aid in healing knee bursitis are vitamin B, vitamin C and vitamin D. Vitamin B and vitamin C are readily available in food, and vitamin D is naturally produced when the body is exposed to sunlight. Taking too much of any vitamin can have side effects, especially if there is a buildup in the body over time. Although vitamin supplements can be very beneficial, it is best to discuss supplementing with vitamins with a healthcare professional.

- **Zinc:** Zinc is a mineral that occurs naturally in the human body and plays a crucial role in cell reproduction, tissue growth and healing wounds. Zinc is vital for healing damaged and infected muscle tissue. Available in capsules and tablets, the recommended dosage is 10mg per day. Check the packaging to see how much needs to be taken daily to reach the recommended dosage.

8.2 Complementary Treatments

There are complementary treatments available that can successfully treat knee bursitis. Complimentary treatments are usually most successful when combined with other treatment. For people who cannot, or would prefer not to take strong pharmaceutical drugs, complementary treatments combined with natural remedies and supplements can be very successful in treating knee pain and in healing knee bursitis. The exception is always septic knee bursitis, that requires immediate antibiotic treatment. Once the infection has cleared, the patient can consider complimentary treatments to facilitate healing.

Acupuncture

Acupuncture is an ancient complementary medical practice that was developed in China. It is discussed in depth in ancient Chinese medical texts that date back to around 475 BC to 221 BC. These texts are regarded as the fundamental doctrinal source of Traditional Chinese medicine. Early explores made mention of acupuncture as a medical treatment from the early 1600's, but it was not explored as a medical treatment until the early 1800's, when European physicians started to study acupuncture and the effects it had on patients. Still, acupuncture was paid little attention and remained relatively unknown in the Western world until the early 1970's, when Major general Walter Tkach, a physician to President Richard Nixon of the United States, wrote an article in the Reader's Digest that brought it to the public's attention. Since then, acupuncture has gained momentum as a complementary treatment. Today, many healthcare professionals recommend acupuncture and even refer their patients to acupuncturists for treatment of various medical conditions, and in particular pain control. Many hospitals and healthcare facilities also offer acupuncture.

In 2003, the World Health Organization sanctioned acupuncture when it listed a number of conditions that can be successfully treated. Among the conditions listed by the World Health Organization are conditions that result in chronic skeletal and muscular pain, as well as high blood pressure.

Although high blood pressure is not a symptom of knee bursitis, the stress and anxiety caused by the onset and persistence of severe pain and inflammation can lead to temporary high blood pressure. The stress and anxiety can be relieved by acupuncture and help bring down high blood pressure. Acupuncture can also relieve the pain that is a major symptom of knee bursitis and restore knee mobility.

What to Expect from Acupuncture Treatment

Acupuncture involves inserting very fine needles into the skin at specific points, according to the condition being treated. These points are situated along energy-flow meridians throughout the body. There are 350 acupuncture points throughout the body. There is no scientific proof that the meridians or acupuncture points exist, but there is also no scientific proof that they do not exist. Needles are inserted in different combination that dictates the desired result. Some Western medical experts believe that acupuncture works by stimulating nerve endings, that are situated at points where muscles, connective tissue and nerves can be stimulated. This results in increased blood flow to the area and the body's natural painkillers being stimulated. Most clinical tests that have set out to prove or disprove the value of acupuncture have been inconclusive. Either way, there are healthcare professionals and patients worldwide that believe wholeheartedly in the medical benefits of acupuncture.

On arrival at an acupuncturist's consulting room, a patient will be asked to complete a form listing their personal details and also give details of existing health conditions. Before an acupuncturist begins treatment, they will first examine the patient from head to toe and discuss not only the medical condition to be treated, but the patient's overall health. At this point, both the acupuncturist and the patient should be asking questions and discussing the patient's health freely. Acupuncture looks to not only treat the existing medical condition, but to address underlying causes as well. The acupuncturist will most likely tell the patient what acupuncture meridians and acupuncture points will be treated, and also give an idea of how many acupuncture sessions will be required.

Following that, the patient will be asked to lie down in a position that allows easy access to the relevant meridians and acupuncture points that need to be treated. The area of skin is sanitized and very thin, sterile, single-use, disposable needles are inserted into the skin. The process is almost pain-free. There can be a brief stinging sensation as each needle is inserted, and a brief aching at the base of the needle as it comes to rest in the skin, but many patients report no pain or discomfort. Needles are left in the skin for anywhere from five to thirty minutes, depending on the condition being treated. In that time, the patient is kept warm and comfortable and encouraged to relax. Removal of the needles is painless.

The number of acupuncture treatments required depends on the condition being treated and the patient's overall health condition. Knee bursitis will most likely require two to three treatments a week over a total of about ten sessions.

There are very few side effects of acupuncture, although some patients do experience bruising and pain after a session. In rare cases, patients report muscle spasms and muscle twitching after a session as well. Pain and muscle spasms or twitching usually dissipates within 24 hours of acupuncture treatment. There are also reports of patients experiencing dizziness and even fainting after an acupuncture session, but this is mostly attributed to either getting up too quickly after a treatment or having acupuncture treatment on an empty stomach.

Note: people who suffer from bleeding disorders or who are taking blood thinning medication must not have acupuncture.

Selecting an Acupuncturist

Unfortunately, many countries do not require acupuncturists to be licensed, and where licensing is a requirement the standards vary greatly. It is best to discuss acupuncture with a healthcare professional and ask if they can refer a professional practitioner. Some medical insurers are starting to pay for acupuncture treatment for specific conditions, so medical insurers would be able to recommend approved practitioners, even if they do not cover the cost.

Many physical therapists are also trained to practice acupuncture, and no hospital or healthcare centre will allow an untrained or unethical acupuncturist to operate from their premises, so consider where a practitioner's rooms are situated. Select an acupuncturist that has internet visibility and is listed on websites offering medical treatments. Also, ask questions about qualifications when making an appointment, and inspect the rooms carefully on arrival. If the acupuncturist does not use sterile, single-use, disposable needles and wear disposable sterile gloves during treatment, do not proceed.

Chiropractic Treatment

Knee bursitis can be successfully treated by a chiropractor. Adjustments and manipulations of muscles and soft tissue that surround the knee joint help restore normal biomechanics within the knee joint and re-establish knee mobility. Chiropractic is a form of alternative medicine concerned with the diagnosis and treatment of mechanical disorders of the musculoskeletal system, especially the spine and knee.

Chiropractic treatments first saw the light of day when Daniel David Palmer of Iowa in the United States of America opened the first chiropractic school in 1897. The school offered training in vitalism, magnetism, naturalism and spiritualism. The profession was heavily curarized by qualified medical practitioners and labelled as "quackery" for decades, during which there were many legal challenges, and many chiropractors were jailed for practising medicine without a license. Despite this, the chiropractic practice continued to survive and chiropractors treated many patients successfully.

By the 1930's, chiropractic was the most popular treatment in the United States and there were over 25,000 practising chiropractors across the country. Despite early struggles for survival, by the mid-1970's the chiropractic profession began organizing itself into professional bodies that were aligned with each other, and by the mid-1990's, a growing scholarly interest in chiropractic aided efforts to establish clinical guidelines and improve service quality.

Today, chiropractors have to undergo extensive training in chiropractic care at registered training facilities. On graduation, they become licensed practitioners. Chiropractors have to renew their license to practice at time intervals determined by the country and state where they practice. Chiropractors do not hold a medical degree and they are not medical doctors. Although a qualified chiropractor is given the title of Doctor of Chiropractic, they are not licensed to write medical prescriptions or perform surgery. In most instances, chiropractors work closely with healthcare professionals and medical physicians to determine what treatments are required to reduce a patient's pain and speed up the healing process.

What to Expect from Chiropractic Treatment

On arrival at a chiropractor's consulting rooms, a patient will be asked to complete a form listing their personal details and also give details of existing health conditions. Before a chiropractor begins treatment, they will first examine the patient from head to toe and discuss not only the medical condition to be treated but the patient's overall health. A thorough chiropractic exam includes general tests such as blood pressure, pulse, respiration, and reflexes, as well as specific orthopaedic and neurological tests. Special attention will be paid to the range of motion and muscle strength and tone of the affected knee joint. At this point, both the chiropractor and the patient should be asking questions and discussing the patient's health freely. Chiropractic looks to not only treat the existing medical condition, but to address underlying causes as well. The chiropractor will advise the patient if any further diagnostic procedures are required. A chiropractor can request X-rays, an MRI scan or laboratory tests from outside medical facilities. If a patient has been referred by a healthcare professional, these diagnostic procedures might already have been conducted and the results made available to the chiropractor. After that, the chiropractor will tell the patient what chiropractic treatments will work best and also give an idea of how many chiropractic treatments will be required. Some chiropractors will give the diagnosis and recommended treatment to a patient in writing, so that the patient can discuss it with their healthcare professional or physician before commencing with treatment. Some patients might also want the diagnosis and estimated cost of treatment to get prior approval from their health insurance plan before starting treatment.

The short-term goal of chiropractic treatment is to reduce knee pain and restore normal muscle balance and knee joint function. The long-term goals include restoring knee function, independence and tolerance of daily activities and knee mobility. A chiropractor uses hands-on treatment methods and chiropractic treatment may include:

- Adjustments to key functions
- Ultrasound, electrical stimulation or traction to improve soft tissue healing and pain control
- Exercises to strengthen and stretch muscles and ligaments to improve muscle balance, strength, and coordination
- Massage and application of heat or cold compresses
- Training methods to improve posture and motor control
- Training methods to reduce anxiety

There are very few side effects of chiropractic treatments, although some patients do experience discomfort in the area treated immediately after a treatment session. In rare cases, patients report pain and discomfort in areas other than the area treated, including headaches. Discomfort and pain usually dissipate within 24 hours of chiropractic treatment. There are also very rare reports of patients experiencing dizziness and nausea after a chiropractic treatment.

Selecting a Chiropractor

Chiropractic treatment has become widely accepted by healthcare professionals, physical therapists and physicians, particularly for treating musculoskeletal conditions (like knee bursitis), so it is easy to get a recommendation or even a referral to a registered chiropractor. Many chiropractors practice from rooms in or close to hospitals or healthcare centres to allow patients easy access to chiropractic treatments. Also, look for a chiropractor that has internet visibility and is listed on websites offering medical treatments. Ask if they are licensed to practice when making an appointment and inspect the rooms carefully on arrival. The rooms must look professional and similar to those of any medical professional. Qualifications and up-to-date licensing must be on public display. Otherwise, patients can ask to view them before commencing treatment.

Other Complementary Treatments

There are other complementary treatments that can help to treat knee bursitis. Most of these treatments are best used as part of the healing and strengthening process, rather than in the first few days of knee bursitis when pain control and rest is recommended.

Applied Kinesiology

A kinesiologist is highly qualified and licensed healthcare professional, who has studied the actions and working of muscles and the movement of the human body. A kinesiologist can identify what is causing imbalances within the body's system and how best to re-establish that balance. Many kinesiologists are also qualified medical doctors, dentists, chiropractors and osteopaths. These healthcare professionals use applied kinesiology in addition to their existing speciality.

Kinesiology is a non-invasive mostly hands-on therapy that aims to determine where imbalances lie in the combined body, mind and spirit. A kinesiologist uses muscle testing and measures of the effects of stress on the neurological areas of the body, like the brain and spinal column, to define and address imbalances.

Reflexology

Reflexology is often mistaken for a foot massage or a spa treatment, which it is not. Reflexology is actually a system of massage used to relieve tension and treat illness, based on the theory that there are reflex points on the feet, hands, and head linked to every part of the body. There is evidence that reflexology was practised in China and Egypt more than 4,000 years ago.

A reflexologist will conduct a health history and explain how reflexology works and what can be expected during a session.

Yoga

Yoga is a Hindu spiritual and ascetic discipline, a part of which (including breath control, simple meditation and the adoption of specific bodily postures) is widely practised for health and relaxation. There are yoga poses that can be beneficial to healing knee bursitis.

Chapter 9: Knee Bursitis Assistive Aids

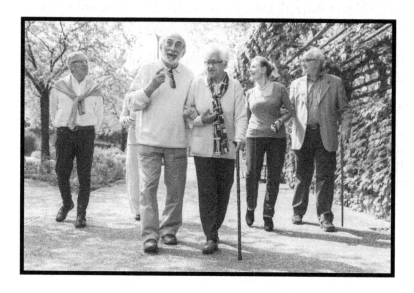

Knee bursitis is a temporary condition that is cleared within about ten days in most healthy people. Irrespective of how long it takes for knee bursitis to heal, the main requirement for successful healing is the rest the knee joint. There are not many orthopaedic assistive aids that will help a person suffering from knee bursitis to heal quicker or become more mobile. The best assistive aids are practical items that compliment walking and resting positions.

It is very important to make some simple safety modifications to the living environment to prevent falls, when using orthopaedic assistive aids. Some points to consider are:

- Removing loose floor throw rugs
- Removing or tying up electrical cords
- Arranging furniture to make clear pathways in and between rooms
- Keeping stairs clear of carpeting and clutter
- Using non-slip bath mats
- Keeping rooms well-lit and installing a nightlight along the route between the bedroom and the bathroom

- Placing items within easy reach and removing unnecessary items

9.1 Walking Sticks

The most successful assistive walking aid for patients suffering from knee bursitis is a walking stick, also known as a trekking stick or walking cane. Branded by many as something outdated and reserved for the elderly, a walking stick is a practical and handy aid for people of all ages. A walking stick is a cost-effective and practical item that can be easily stored away for use at a later time if necessary.

Using a walking stick eases pain from the lower back down to the feet, and greatly reduces stress on joints. Using two walking sticks simultaneously is twice as effective. Although the concept of using two walking sticks might appear strange, hikers regularly use two trekking sticks when covering rough terrain to maintain balance, reduce stress on their joints and prevent injury. Clinical studies have shown that using a walking stick reduces stress on the knee joints by more than 10%. Improved balance is also very important for anyone suffering from knee bursitis because a painful knee causes reduced joint mobility and stability which can lead to a fall. Falling on a knee that is already affected by knee bursitis can complicate the condition and slow down healing, and it can also lead to cuts, bruises, sprains and even broken bones anywhere else on the body.

How to use a Walking Stick

It is vital to choose the correct length of walking stick. When in a standing position, the top of the walking stick should reach the crease on the inside wrist. If using a single walking stick, it must be held in the opposite hand from the knee affected by knee bursitis. For instance, if the right knee is affected, the walking stick must be held in the left hand and if the left knee is affected, the walking stick must be held in the right hand. This helps to stabilize the pelvis and lessen the stress and load on the affected knee joint.

To begin walking, place the walking stick about one small stride ahead and step forward with the unaffected leg. To climb stairs, place the walking stick in the hand opposite the injured leg and use the free hand to hold onto the handrail. Step up with the unaffected leg first and then bring the affected leg up. To come downstairs, place the walking stick on the step first and bring the affected leg down next, followed by the unaffected leg that will carry the full body weight.

9.2 Crutches

Crutches are useful only if the affected knee cannot carry any weight at all. Walking safely and comfortably with crutches can be difficult to master and can become painful on the arms. Only choose crutches as a walking aid if it is absolutely necessary.

How to use a Crutches

It is vital to choose the correct length of crutch. When in a standing position, the top of each crutch should reach 1 to 2 inches (2.5 to 5cm) below each armpit and the grips of each crutch should be even with the hipline. Elbows should be bent slightly when holding the handgrips. To avoid damage to the blood vessels and nerve endings in the armpits, the weight must be placed on the hands via the handgrips and not on the underarm supports.

To begin walking, lean forward slightly and place both crutches about one stride ahead. Begin the first step as if it is to be on the affected leg but shift the weight to the crutches instead. Slowly bring the body forward and between the crutches. Make the next step with the unaffected leg. Once the unaffected leg is firmly on the ground, move both crutches forward again at the same time to take the next step. Make sure to keep the eyes straight ahead and not to look down at the feet in order to keep balanced.

To sit when using crutches, choose a solid and sturdy chair that will not move. Place the affected leg in front and move both crutches to one hand. Use the other hand to feel behind for the chair and slowly lower the body into the chair. Once seated, lean the crutches securely close by, so that they do not fall over. To stand up, side forward to the front of the chair and take both crutches in the same hand as the affected leg. Push the body up on the unaffected leg while leaning on the crutches.

To climb and descend stairs with crutches, the patient must be strong and flexible. A frail patient or a patient that is still weak from convalescence (especially from septic knee bursitis), should avoid climbing stairs on crutches. To climb stairs, face the stairway and hold the handrail with one hand, while tucking both crutches under the armpit of the other side. Lead with the unaffected leg, while keeping the affected leg raised and behind. To descend stairs, keep the affected leg in front, and hop down each step on the unaffected leg, taking one step at a time.

9.3 Orthopaedic Cushions

A patient suffering from knee bursitis will have pain when they sit and move around and this is where orthopaedic cushions can be of great help. Orthopaedic cushions are designed to relieve pressure on joints, while promoting healthy blood circulation. They are available in different shapes, thickness and designed to carry different body weights. It is best to get professional advice when choosing orthopaedic cushion to make sure that the cushions selected do address the patient's specific condition. Physical therapists are most qualified to give sound advice on orthopaedic cushions.

Chapter 10: Natural Remedies for Knee Bursitis Pain

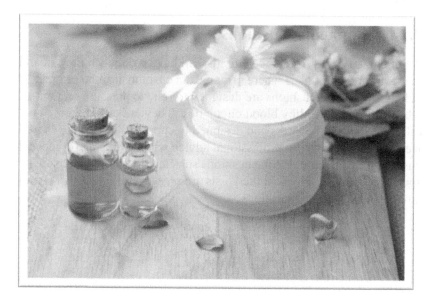

There are a number of natural remedies that can alleviate the pain and inflammation caused by knee bursitis. If fever and flu-like symptoms accompany knee pain, the condition requires immediate medical intervention, because it is most likely septic knee bursitis. Natural remedies cannot cure septic knee bursitis and the patient needs antibiotic treatment as soon as possible. Once a patient is being treated with antibiotics and the infection in the knee bursa is under control, natural remedies can aid healing as long as they have been cleared by a healthcare professional.

The following natural remedies can be self-managed at home and the elements used can be bought from most supermarkets and pharmacies.

10.1 Natural Remedies

1. **Apple Cider Vinegar**

   Apple cider vinegar helps to restore alkalinity in the body and that aids in reducing inflammation. Apple cider vinegar also contains minerals like calcium, phosphorus and potassium, that help balance body fluids. There are two ways to use apple cider vinegar to treat knee bursitis:

- Soak a face cloth or thin absorbent pad in undiluted apple cider vinegar and place it directly on the affected area of the knee joint. If possible, wrap it to secure it well. Keep it secured over the affected area for a few hours or overnight. Use daily but stop use immediately, if there are any signs of skin irritation.
- Place one tablespoon of undiluted apple cider vinegar together with a teaspoon of raw honey in a glass of warm water. Drink as a tonic twice a day. Always use raw honey, because it has natural anti-inflammatory and antibiotic properties, while in processed honey and runny-honey these properties are lost.

Note: people with diseases of the gastrointestinal tract, like stomach ulcers, ingest apple cider vinegar with caution, because it can aggravate the gastrointestinal tract.

2. Capsicum Frutescens
Capsicum frutescens is the highly purified, heat-producing component in chilli peppers. It can be bought in gel or cream format and also as a patch. Capsicum frutescens activates nerve receptors in the skin causing heat, stinging or itching sensations. Prolonged activation of these nerve receptors causes them to lose their ability to function properly and to process pain signals for extended periods of time. Capsicum frutescens must not be used regularly to keep the nerve receptors from working properly and processing pain signals. Use the treatment three times a day for only a short period.
Note: capsicum frutescens can irritate sensitive skins. If it does, stop using it immediately.

3. Castor Oil
Ricinoleic acid in castor oil has anti-inflammatory properties that aid in reducing pain and minimizing inflammation caused by knee bursitis. Castor oil also helps improve knee joint mobility.

It is important to note that castor oil is a natural laxative, so it must not be ingested to treat knee bursitis. Use castor oil externally:
- Soak an absorbent cloth or pad in castor oil
- Lie down and elevate the affected leg to a comfortable position that is above the level of the heart
- Use pillows to keep the leg comfortably elevated

- Place it directly over the affected area of the knee joint and secure it with a protective waterproof wrap
- Place a hot water bottle or warm compress over the same area of the affected knee
- Keep both the castor oil and the warm compress over the affected knee area for 30 to 40 minutes
- After removal, gently massage the castor oil residue into the skin
- After the massage, keep the leg elevated and rested for at least another 15 minutes
- Use this treatment once a day

Note: avoid massage in cases of septic knee bursitis. Rather, gently wipe the castor oil residue off the skin with a warm cloth.

4. Cold Compress

Cold compresses aid in reducing pain by numbing the affected area and help in bringing down swelling. They are most effective when used in the first 24 to 48 hours after symptoms first began.

Most pharmacies sell cold compresses that can be kept in a freezer, or a cold compress can be made by wrapping a few ice cubes in a thin towel. Use cold compresses as follows:

- Lie down and elevate the affected leg to a comfortable position that is above the level of the heart
- Use pillows to keep the leg comfortably elevated
- Place the cold compress over the affected knee joint and keep it there for up to 15 minutes at a time
- After removing the cold compress, keep the leg elevated and rested for at least another 15 minutes
- Repeat the process a few times a day until there is relief

Note: never apply ice or an unprotected icepack directly to the skin, because it will damage the skin.

5. Kinesiology Tape

Kinesiology taping is a form of sports taping that encourages the lymphatic and circulatory systems to flow and work efficiently through the specific placement of strips of kinesiology tape. It also adds in reducing pain and swelling. When applied correctly to the knee area, kinesiology tape can increase joint stability and support the surrounding muscles. Kinesiology tape is available from sports outlets and physical therapists.

6. Warm Compress

Warm compresses are usually more beneficial to knee bursitis patients and can be used to alleviate symptoms for as long as the knee bursitis perseveres. A warm compress improves blood flow in the affected knee joint, reduces stiffness in the knee joint and soothes inflammation.

Most pharmacies sell warm compresses that can be warmed in a microwave, as well as electric heating pads. A hot water bottle also works well, or a warm compress can be made by soaking a towel with hot (not boiling) water and wringing the towel out well. Use warm compresses as follows:
- Lie down and elevate the affected leg to a comfortable position that is above the level of the heart
- Use pillows to keep the leg comfortably elevated
- Place the warm compress over the affected knee joint and keep it there for 15 to 20 minutes at a time
- After removing the warm compress, keep the leg elevated and rested for at least another 15 minutes
- Repeat the process a few times a day until there is relief

Note: a few drops of essential oil can be added to the hot water before dampening the towel. Essential oils are covered further on in this chapter.

7. Dimethyl Sulfoxide

Dimethyl sulfoxide is derived from wood pulp and is available in liquid and gel form from most pharmacies. If used as a topical analgesic, it easily penetrates the skin to bring relief from pain and swelling and speed up the healing process. Pharmaceutical grade dimethyl sulfoxide comes in different grades, i.e. 99.9%, 80%, 70%, 50% and 25%. To treat knee bursitis, it is best to use a 70% solution, as follows:
- Soak a cotton ball with dimethyl sulfoxide and apply to the affected knee joint
- Rub gently onto the skin until all the dimethyl sulfoxide is absorbed
- Use the dimethyl sulfoxide rub up to three times a day

Note: dimethyl sulfoxide naturally feels warm on the skin, but if there are any signs of skin irritation, clean the area thoroughly and stop use. If there are no improvements after using dimethyl sulfoxide two or three times, also stop using it.

8. Ginger

Ginger has natural pain relieving and anti-inflammatory properties that can help reduce the pain, inflammation and discomfort caused by knee bursitis. Ginger also improves blood circulation that promotes healing. Fresh ginger is readily available and is best, because none of the healing properties have been compromised by processing. Also, pure ginger essential oils work well as a massage oil but must not be ingested. Fresh ginger can be used in two ways.

As a compress:

- Grate 3 to 4 tablespoons of fresh ginger and place it in an unbleached natural cloth
- Tie the cloth tightly and steep the ginger in hot water for 30 seconds to draw out the natural oils
- Lie down and elevate the affected leg to a comfortable position that is above the level of the heart
- Use pillows to keep the leg comfortably elevated
- Cool cloth until it is comfortable to the touch and then place it directly on the affected area of the knee
- Leave it on for 10 to 15 minutes
- After removing the cold compress, keep the leg elevated and rested for at least another 15 minutes
- Repeat the process a few times a day until there is relief

As a drink:

Gently boil one tablespoon of sliced fresh ginger in two cups of water for ten minutes. Put aside to cool. Strain to remove the ginger and add one teaspoon of raw honey. Always use raw honey because it has natural anti-inflammatory and antibiotic properties. Drink as a tea three times a day.

9. White Willow Bark

White willow bark contains salicin - a compound produced naturally in the bark that acts as an anti-inflammatory agent when ingested. It is very effective for treating knee bursitis because it works as a natural pain killer while reducing inflammation and swelling. White willow bark is available from health shops and pharmacies. Use it as a drink by adding half a teaspoon white willow bark to a cup of boiling water. Cover and allow it to steep for 15 minutes. Strain and add one teaspoon of raw honey. Drink as a tea twice a day.

Note: while willow bark is not suitable for people taking blood-thinning medication.

10.2 Massage

Massage improves circulation and reduces the swelling and stiffness in the knee joint caused by knee bursitis. Massage also promotes effective relaxation. A massage oil must always be used to prevent damage to the skin. Massage oil can be of a single type of oil known as a carrier oil or a blend of carrier oil and specific essential oils, that are used to relieve pain and inflammation. Massage oils are most effective if the skin has been warmed up with a cloth steeped in warm water just before application, or if the oil has been warmed before application. The oil can be warmed by keeping the sealed container in a bowl of warm water for a few minutes before use.

Certain carrier oils also have properties that will aid in alleviating the discomfort caused by knee bursitis and in healing knee bursitis. These carrier oils are:

- Castor oil: ricinoleic acid in castor oil has anti-inflammatory properties that aid in reducing pain and minimizing inflammation caused by knee bursitis.
- Coconut oil: it has anti-inflammatory and analgesic properties that help to reduce pain. It also helps to reduce topical inflammation, which is very helpful if the knee bursitis is accompanied by bruising.
- Extra virgin olive oil: helps to reduce pain and inflammation, making it ideal for treating knee bursitis. It is important to use olive oil that is for massage, and not for consumption. Olive oil used in the kitchen has a much thicker consistency than olive oil produced for massage.
- Jojoba oil: it is very close to the oils naturally produced by the skin. It helps to reduce inflammation and allows topical preparation to be absorbed more easily.

10.3 Essential Oils

Essential oils are very potent and must never be applied directly to the skin and never be ingested. Only a few drops of essential oil must be used for each massage. Essential oils are always diluted in a neutral carrier oil, and for pain relief the best ratio is four drops of essential oil to every tablespoon of carrier oil. Make sure that all the massage oils being used are pure and not synthetic, because synthetic oils have no healing properties and contain artificial chemical fragrances. Synthetic oils also in some instances contain artificial coloring, that can cause damage to the skin surface and potential allergic reactions once absorbed into the skin.

To make a massage oil for topical pain relief of knee bursitis, it is best to use a small glass bottle with a lid that seals tightly. Dilute four drops of the selected essential oil in a tablespoon of carrier oil, such as castor oil, coconut oil, jojoba oil or olive oil. Shake well to mix thoroughly and remember to gently warm the oil mix before applying to the skin.

It is important to note that certain essential oils will stain fabric, so caution must be taken to protect bed linen and clothing.

There are many essential oils that have healing properties and provide relief from pain and inflammation. Many essential oils also promote relaxation by calming the nerves under the skin. Different types of essential oil can be combined to benefit from the various properties each oil brings to treat knee bursitis. The ratio of four drops of essential oil to one tablespoon of carrier oil must not be exceeded, even when blending different essential oils with a carrier oil. Essential and carrier oils are absorbed into the skin and from there into the bloodstream, so the affected area of the knee must not be massaged more than once a day. If there is any negative reaction during or after the massage, stop immediately and rinse all the oils off the skin with a warm facecloth. Do not use the same oils again. Essential oils must never be applied to broken skin or an open wound.

The following essential oils provide relief for knee bursitis:

1. Arnica

Arnica essential oil is a potent oil that is especially effective for treating inflammation and muscle damage. It also improves blood circulation and aids in transporting blood and other fluids that are accumulated in the area of the knee bursae away to speed up the healing process.

2. **Bergamot**

   Bergamot essential oil contains analgesic elements that help to relieve pain and reduce stress and anxiety. It works by reducing nerve sensitivity to pain and in so doing easing the pain. Also, inhalation of bergamot essential oil during massage has an overall calming effect. This is due to certain calming hormones in the body being triggered by inhalation.

3. **Black Pepper**

   Black pepper essential oil is a potent oil used to relieve muscle aches and pain. It also improves blood circulation to reduce inflammation. Black pepper essential oil also contains antibacterial elements.

4. **Chamomile**

   Chamomile essential oil contains analgesic elements that help to relieve pain and reduce stress and anxiety. It works particularly well on inflamed joints and muscles by reducing inflammation and soothing the muscles. Chamomile essential oil has a soothing and calming effect on the whole body. Flavonoids in chamomile essential oil are absorbed into the skin and from there into the bloodstream, allowing it to not only soothe the area where it is being applied but to also travel through the body. The calming and relaxing effects of chamomile essential oil can also be experienced through inhalation.

5. **Clary Sage**

   Clary sage essential oil contains analgesic elements that relax muscles and relieve muscle cramps. It also has a calming effect on the mind.

6. **Eucalyptus**

   Eucalyptus essential oil is a powerful oil that contains elements that help to get rid of nerve-related pain and discomfort. It has anti-oxidant, anti-inflammatory and antibacterial compounds. Inhaling eucalyptus essential oil can help relieve pain and lower blood pressure as well. Eucalyptus essential oil is best known for its ability to relieve pain and inflammation caused by sinus and chest infections, but it is very effective in treating joint and muscle pain as well.

7. **Frankincense**

   Frankincense essential oil contains elements that block enzymes connected with inflammation. It also has pain relieving analgesic properties and aids in relaxing muscle tension.

8. **Ginger**

   Ginger essential oil alleviates joint pain and eases stiffness in the knee muscles due to its anti-inflammatory and analgesic properties.

9. **Helichrysum**

   Helichrysum essential oil has powerful pain-relieving properties and elements that help repair damaged skin and tissue. It is an anti-inflammatory and analgesic oil that can relieve chronic pain by reducing enzymes related to inflammation, eliminating free radicals and reducing swelling. Helichrysum essential oil has been shown to not only heal bruising, but also prevent bruising if it is applied while bruising is taking place.

10. **Juniper**

    Juniper essential oil contains an element that relieves pain and stiffness in the muscles of the knee joint. It has a numbing effect on the pain that has been backed up by numerous studies.

11. **Lavender**

    Lavender is undoubtedly the best known and most widely used essential oil for pain relief. Lavender essential oil contains compounds that have been proven to act as a mild sedative and reduce stress and anxiety. It also contains elements that reduce inflammation and have an analgesic effect. Inhaling lavender essential oil also offers the benefit of relieving pain and reducing stress and anxiety. Also, inhalation encourages restful sleep.

    Lavender essential oil is one of the few essential oils that is mild enough to apply directly to the skin without dilution in a carrier oil. Always use caution; it is best to apply lavender essential oil directly to a very small patch of skin first and wait for 24 hours to see if there is a negative reaction.

12. **Lemongrass**

    Lemongrass essential oil is a refreshing oil that contains elements that relieve pain, reduce inflammation and enhance the mood. It inhibits inflammatory responses in the body by blocking inflammatory related enzymes.

13. **Peppermint**

    Peppermint essential oil contains analgesic, anti-inflammatory, anti-spasmodic and anti-microbial elements. It can successfully treat minor fungal infections and is well known as a natural decongestant for treating sinus and chest conditions. Peppermint essential oil has a cooling effect on the skin.

14. **Rose Geranium**

    Rose geranium essential oil is primarily anti-inflammatory, but also has analgesic properties. It soothes nerve endings to ease pain and discomfort.

15. Rosemary

Rosemary essential oil contains powerful anti-inflammatory elements and also elements that improve blood circulation to facilitate healing. It also contains elements that relieve muscle pain and spasms. Rosemary essential oil is excellent for treating the symptoms of knee bursitis and works well with pharmaceutical drugs to speed up recovery.

16. Sandalwood

Sandalwood essential oil contains anti-inflammatory and analgesic elements that ease joint pain and facilitate healing. It also has powerful elements that sedate the nervous system and inhibits the production of adrenalin. Inhaling sandalwood essential oil has a relaxing effect.

17. Sweet Marjoram

Sweet marjoram essential oil contains anti-inflammatory and sedative elements and is known to relieve chronic pain, including a toothache.

18. Thyme

Thyme essential oil contains anti-inflammatory and analgesic elements. It successfully suppresses enzymes related to inflammation and can be used for chronic pain.

19. Vetiver

Vetiver essential oil contains anti-inflammatory elements and also elements that improve blood circulation and soothe the nervous system. Vetiver essential oil brings general relief to the pain and discomfort caused by knee bursitis.

20. Wintergreen

Wintergreen essential oil contains elements that have been scientifically proven to be similar to aspirin. It is a natural analgesic that successfully treats pain.

21. Yarrow

Yarrow essential oil contains anti-inflammatory and anti-spasmodic elements. It is known to reduce inflammation and successfully treat muscle cramps and spasms.

If massage is not possible, a few drops of any essential oil or a combination of essential oils can also be added to warm bath water and the patient can soak in warm water. The warm bath water opens the pores of the skin and makes absorption of the essential oils through the skin more effective. It is very important to test the essential oils on the patient's skin before the patient soaks in the bath. This can be done by diluting a drop of the essential oil in a few drops of hot water or carrier oil. Soak a cotton ball in the dilution and dab a small amount onto a sensitive area of the patient's skin, like the inner forearm or on the neck. Leave the dilution on the skin and monitor every few hours to see if there are any signs of skin irritation. If there are, rinse the area of skin thoroughly with warm water and wipe clean with a warm facecloth. Do not use that type of essential oil again. Test a different oil in the same way, because if someone has a skin reaction to one type of essential oil, it does not mean that they will react to all types. Three or four essential oils can safely be tested simultaneously in this way as long as a note is made of which oil has been dabbed on what area of the skin; note it down as it is being done.

Essential oils can also be added to the hot water used to make a warm compress by putting a few drops of essential oil into the hot water used before soaking the towel.

Essential oils also work very well when blended into an aqueous cream. It is vital that the ratio of essential oil to aqueous cream is closely measured. Keep the blend at the same ratio as for a carrier oil: four drops of essential oil to one tablespoon of aqueous cream. Ensure that the essential oil is blended very well into the aqueous cream before application. Aqueous creams are easily absorbed into the skin without vigorous rubbing.

10.4 Essential Oil Recipes

You've already learned about the essential oils used for treating knee bursitis, but you may still be nervous about trying it for yourself. If you'd like to give essential oils a try, you'll find some simple recipes in this chapter. These recipes will allow you to use your pain-relieving essential oils in various forms, such as cream, balm, gel, lotion, etc.

The recipes are made with all-natural ingredients you can find online or at your local health food store and they are safe and simple to prepare. Try one or try them all! Here's a list of the essential oil home remedies you'll find in this chapter:

- Peppermint Cold Compress
- Aloe Vera Eucalyptus Gel for Pain
- Rosemary Ginger Balm

- Whipped Wintergreen Body Butter
- Warm Lavender Oil Rub
- Arnica Anti-Inflammatory Cream
- Soothing Eucalyptus Salve
- Frankincense Hot Compress
- Coconut Lemongrass Body Butter
- Healing Chamomile Balm
- Lavender Eucalyptus Liniment
- Pain-Relieving Rose Cream
- Simple Anti-Inflammatory Ointment
- Homemade Hot Pepper Cream
- Cooling Aloe Vera Lotion

To get the most out of these recipes, be sure to purchase high-quality ingredients. Look for 100% pure essential oils and organic additives, such as shea butter, cocoa butter, coconut oil and various carrier oils. When preparing these recipes, you can feel free to customize them according to your preference by swapping out one of the essential oils for another from the list provided earlier in this chapter. So, without further ado, here are the recipes!

Peppermint Cold Compress

Ingredients:

- 2 cups cold water
- 3 drops peppermint essential oil
- 6 ice cubes

Instructions:

1. Stir the peppermint essential oil into the cold water.
2. Add the ice cubes and let them dissolve, stirring occasionally until they melt.
3. Soak a clean cloth or hand towel in the liquid.
4. Wring out the excess moisture then apply to the affected knee.

Aloe Vera Eucalyptus Gel for Pain

Ingredients:

- ½ cup 100% pure Aloe Vera gel
- 20 drops eucalyptus essential oil

- 10 drops wintergreen essential oil

Instructions:

1. Combine the Aloe Vera gel and essential oils in a small glass mixing bowl.
2. Stir until well combined then transfer to a dark glass bottle or a small glass jar.
3. Apply the mixture liberally to the affected area.
4. Massage the gel into the skin until it is well absorbed.

Rosemary Ginger Balm

Ingredients:

- 1 cup jojoba oil
- 1 ounce (30 grams) grated beeswax
- 5 drops rosemary essential oil
- 5 drops eucalyptus essential oil
- 3 drops ginger essential oil

Instructions:

1. Combine the beeswax and jojoba oil in a double boiler over low heat.
2. Heat until the beeswax is melted then stir smooth.
3. Remove from heat and whisk in the essential oils until well combined.
4. Pour into small glass jars and cover with the lids.
5. Let rest at room temperature until the balm solidifies then use.

Whipped Wintergreen Body Butter

Ingredients:

- ½ cup organic shea butter
- ½ cup organic coconut oil
- 3 tablespoons sweet almond oil
- ¼ cup magnesium oil
- 25 drops wintergreen essential oil

Instructions:

1. Combine the shea butter, coconut oil and sweet almond oil in a double boiler over low heat.
2. Heat until the oils are melted then stir smooth.

3. Remove from heat and transfer to the fridge – cool for 45 to 60 minutes until it hardens slightly.
4. Beat the mixture with a hand mixer on the medium-high speed setting.
5. Add the magnesium oil, a tablespoon at a time, then beat in the wintergreen essential oil.
6. Beat for 2 to 3 minutes until the mixture is light and fluffy.
7. Transfer to a glass jar and cover with the lid then chill for 30 to 60 minutes until it hardens slightly. Use as desired.

Warm Lavender Oil Rub

Ingredients:

- ½ tablespoon extra-virgin olive oil
- 10 drops lavender essential oil

Instructions:

1. Heat the olive oil in the microwave until very warm but not hot.
2. Stir in the lavender essential oil.
3. Rub the oil into the skin on your affected knee.
4. Massage the area until the oil is well absorbed.

Arnica Anti-Inflammatory Cream

Ingredients:

- ¾ cup sweet almond oil
- ½ cup dried arnica flowers
- 5 tablespoons grated beeswax
- ¼ cup organic shea butter
- ¼ teaspoon borax
- ¼ cup filtered water

Instructions:

1. Combine the sweet almond oil and dried arnica flowers in a saucepan over low heat.
2. Heat for about 30 minutes until warm then strain the mixture into a bowl, discarding the solids.
3. Return the oil to the saucepan then add the beeswax and heat until the wax is melted.
4. Stir in the shea butter until well combined.

5. In a separate saucepan, whisk the borax into the water and heat until steaming.
6. Slowly pour the borax mixture into the oil, stirring constantly.
7. Stir until the two mixtures become one, using a hand mixer if needed.
8. Transfer to a glass jar and cover with the lid.
9. Apply the cream to the affected area and rub it in well.

Soothing Eucalyptus Salve

Ingredients:

- ½ cup sweet almond oil
- ½ cup organic grapeseed oil
- 2 tablespoons grated beeswax
- 2 vitamin E oil capsules
- 10 drops eucalyptus essential oil
- 5 drops lavender essential oil
- 5 drops frankincense essential oil

Instructions:

1. Combine the sweet almond oil, grapeseed oil and beeswax in a double boiler over low heat.
2. Heat until the beeswax is melted then stir smooth.
3. Remove from heat and stir in the vitamin E oil then set aside to cool for 5 minutes.
4. Add the essential oils and stir well.
5. Pour into a glass jar and cover with the lid – let rest for 2 hours.
6. Apply the mixture to the affected area and rub it in well.

Frankincense Hot Compress

Ingredients:

- 1 cup water
- 10 drops frankincense essential oil

Instructions:

1. Heat the water on the stove until it is hot, but not too hot to touch.
2. Remove from heat then add the frankincense essential oil.
3. Soak a cloth or small hand towel in the mixture then wring out the excess moisture.

4. Apply the hot compress to the affected area.

Coconut Lemongrass Body Butter

Ingredients:

- ½ cup organic shea butter
- ½ cup organic cocoa butter
- ½ cup organic coconut oil
- ½ cup jojoba oil
- 20 drops lemongrass essential oil

Instructions:

1. Combine the shea butter, cocoa butter, coconut oil and jojoba oil in a double boiler over low heat.
2. Heat until the ingredients are melted then stir smooth.
3. Remove from heat and stir in the lemongrass essential oil.
4. Let cool to room temperature then beat with a hand mixer until light and fluffy.
5. Spoon into a glass jar then cover with the lid and store at room temperature.

Healing Chamomile Balm

Ingredients:

- ¼ cup organic coconut oil
- ¼ cup jojoba oil
- 1 tablespoon grated beeswax
- 1 vitamin E oil capsule
- 4 drops chamomile essential oil
- 2 drops lavender essential oil
- 2 drops lemongrass essential oil

Instructions:

1. Combine the coconut oil, jojoba oil and beeswax in a double boiler over medium-low heat.
2. Heat until the coconut oil and beeswax are melted then remove from heat and stir smooth.
3. Stir in the vitamin E oil and the essential oils.
4. Pour the mixture into a small glass jar and cool to room temperature.
5. Cover with the lid and store at room temperature.

6. Use as needed by rubbing into the affected area.

Lavender Eucalyptus Liniment

Ingredients:

- 2 ounces (60 grams) jojoba oil
- 2 ounces (60 grams) sweet almond oil
- 10 drops lavender essential oil
- 10 drops eucalyptus essential oil
- 5 drops rosemary essential oil
- 3 drops ginger essential oil

Instructions:

1. Combine the jojoba oil and sweet almond oil in a small dark glass bottle or jar.
2. Add the essential oils and shake well.
3. Apply a small amount to the affected area and rub it in.

Pain-Relieving Rose Cream

Ingredients:

- ½ cup organic coconut oil
- ½ tablespoon grated beeswax
- 5 drops camphor oil
- 5 drops peppermint essential oil
- 5 drops rose essential oil

Instructions:

1. Combine the coconut oil and beeswax in a double boiler over low heat until melted, then stir smooth.
2. Remove from heat and let the mixture cool for a few minutes then add the camphor oil, peppermint oil and rose essential oil.
3. Stir well then pour into a glass jar and cool completely at room temperature.
4. Apply the cream to the affected area and rub it in well.

Simple Anti-Inflammatory Ointment

Ingredients:

- ½ cup organic coconut oil
- 20 drops frankincense essential oil

- 20 drops sweet marjoram essential oil
- 10 drops ginger essential oil

Instructions:

1. Warm the coconut oil in the microwave until softened.
2. Whisk in the essential oils until well combined.
3. Spoon the mixture into a small glass jar and let rest at room temperature until it starts to solidify.
4. Apply a small amount to the affected area and rub it in well.

Homemade Hot Pepper Cream

Ingredients:

- 3 tablespoons cayenne
- 1 cup extra-virgin olive oil
- ½ cup grated beeswax
- 3 drops black pepper essential oil

Instructions:

1. Whisk the cayenne into the olive oil in a double boiler over medium-low heat.
2. Heat for 10 minutes, stirring often, then stir in the beeswax.
3. Let the mixture sit until the beeswax is melted then stir everything together until well combined.
4. Chill for 10 minutes then add the essential oil and whisk well.
5. Return the mixture to the fridge and chill for another 10 to 15 minutes, then beat with a hand mixer until thick and creamy.
6. Spoon into a glass jar and cover with the lid.
7. Store in the refrigerator for up to 1 ½ weeks, using as needed.

Cooling Aloe Vera Lotion

Ingredients:

- ½ cup organic coconut oil
- ¼ cup organic cocoa butter
- ¼ cup 100% pure Aloe Vera gel
- ½ teaspoon Manuka honey
- 5 drops ylang ylang essential oil
- 4 drops bergamot essential oil
- 1 vitamin E capsule
- 1 tablespoon rose water

Instructions:

1. Combine the cocoa butter and coconut oil in a double boiler over low heat until they are melted.
2. Remove from heat then whisk in the Aloe Vera gel and honey.
3. Chill for 15 minutes until it starts to solidify.
4. Stir in the ylang ylang and bergamot essential oils along with the vitamin E.
5. Beat with a hand mixer until thick and creamy.
6. Chill for 10 minutes then beat again, adding the rose water a little at a time, until light and fluffy.
7. Spoon into a glass jar and store at room temperature.

Chapter 11: Food and Knee Bursitis

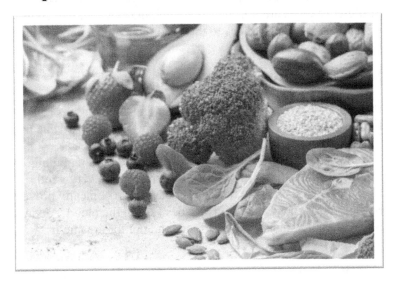

Aseptic knee bursitis in the most common type of knee bursitis, which is an inflammatory condition. Septic knee bursitis is an inflammatory condition that has become infected with bacteria as well. There are many foods that promote inflammation, and many foods that have anti-inflammatory properties. Treatment for any health condition should be looked at from a holistic perspective rather than just relying on pharmaceutical drugs to relieve the symptoms and treat the condition. Very often, lifestyle choices influence a person's health, but many people overlook this fact.

In a world of fast results, fast food, disposable products with instant replacements and emphasized time urgency, most people are unaware that the human body has its own intelligence and timing and that all humans are inextricably connected to cycles of nature and the cycles of the universe. The loss of this ancient wisdom, particularly in the Western World, has resulted in people not knowing what is best for them and desperately turning to pharmaceuticals and quick chemical cures in times of illness. Pharmaceutical drugs and medical procedures most certainly have their place but learning to adopt a more balanced and healthy lifestyle that is in tune with the cycles of nature and the cycles of the universe will make healing easier and lessen the potential for disease in future.

Learning which foods can help to alleviate the symptoms (and potentially the recurrence) of knee bursitis can seem intimidating at first, but if diet changes are introduced slowly, the new diet will soon become palatable and the changes to the meal plan will become a way of life.

11.1 Foods that Alleviate Knee Bursitis

Foods that alleviate any type of bursitis, including knee bursitis have anti-inflammatory properties, because they are high in antioxidants that reduce the damage caused by inflammation. Considering that inflammation is at the heart of almost all health condition, including high amounts of foods that discourage inflammation is a very good option. Most of the foods listed below also have been clinically proven to lower cholesterol and reduce triglycerides (fat) in the blood. Always buy fresh food, rather than processed food, and opt for organic if possible.

Healthy foods should replace the existing diet rather than complement it but if the diet changes seem too extreme, opt to eliminate at least two unhealthy foods (and keep them eliminated) per day and introduce two healthy foods in their place. In that way, the diet changes are more gradual, and new ways of eating should be in place within a week or two.

Avoid over-boiling or deep-frying food and rather opt for steaming, baking or dry-frying cooking methods. Eat at least four to five servings of vegetables per day, three to four servings of fruit per day, one to two servings of beans and legumes per day and five to seven servings of healthy fats per day. Limit each animal protein type to only one to two servings per week. Herbs and spices can be used freely and drink plenty of pure water every day.

The following **vegetables** have known anti-inflammatory properties:

- Allium vegetables:
  - Asparagus
  - Chives
  - Garlic
  - Leeks
  - Onions
  - Scallions
  - Shallots

- Beans and legumes
  - Anasazi beans
  - Adzuki beans
  - Black beans
  - Black-eyed beans
  - Kidney beans
  - Pinto beans
  - Chickpeas
  - Green peas
  - Black-eyed peas
  - Lentils
- Cruciferous green vegetables
  - Bok choy
  - Broccoli
  - Brussels sprouts
  - Cabbage
  - Cauliflower
  - Cress
- Dark leafy green vegetables
  - Collard greens
  - Kale
  - Mustard greens
  - Romaine lettuce
  - Spinach
  - Swiss chard
  - Turnip greens
- Hot peppers
- Nuts and seeds
  - Walnuts, pecan nuts, chestnuts, almonds and hazelnuts have the highest antioxidant content, particularly when the thin skin coating is left intact
  - Chia seeds, flax seeds, hemp seeds, pumpkin seeds, sesame seeds and sunflower seeds
- Root vegetables
  - Beetroot
  - Carrots
  - Parsnip
  - Radish
  - Sweet potato
  - Turnips
- Squash

- o Summer squash (patty pan, zucchini and any type of baby squash)
- o Winter squash (full grown squash with a tough exterior and full-grown seeds inside)
- Vegetable sprouts (any type of young vegetable sprouts)

The following **fruits** have known anti-inflammatory properties:

- Apple
- Apricot
- Blackberries
- Blueberries
- Cherries
- Cranberries
- Cucumber
- Grapes – red and darker skinned only
- Mango
- Nectarine
- Orange
- Pear
- Grapefruit
  - o Pink grapefruit
  - o Red grapefruit
- Papaya
- Pineapple
- Plums
- Pomegranate
- Strawberries
- Tomato
- Watermelon
- Unsweetened dried fruit

The following **herbs** have known anti-inflammatory properties:

- Basil
- Cilantro
- Lavender
- Oregano
- Parsley
- Rosemary
- Thyme

The following **spices** have known anti-inflammatory properties:

- Cayenne pepper
- Cinnamon
- Clove
- Cumin
- Ginger
- Nutmeg
- Turmeric

The following **natural oils** have known anti-inflammatory properties:

- Avocado oil
- Canola oil (pure)
- Extra virgin olive oil
- Flaxseed oil
- Hazelnut oil
- Hemp seed oil
- Safflower oil (high-oleic)
- Sunflower oil (pure)
- Sesame oil
- Walnut oil

The following **alcoholic and non-alcoholic beverages** have known anti-inflammatory properties:

- Chocolate – made with pure dark chocolate
- Tea – limited to four cups per day
  - Ginger tea
  - Green tea
  - Oolong tea
- Wine – organic red wine limited to one or two glasses per day

The following **animal proteins** have known anti-inflammatory properties:

- Eggs
- Fatty cold-water fish
  - Anchovies
  - Herring
  - Mackerel
  - Salmon
  - Sardines

- Organic poultry
- Organic yogurt
- Seafood - fresh

11.2 Foods that Aggravate Knee Bursitis

Foods that aggravate knee bursitis are foods that aggravate existing inflammation or cause inflammation. Clinical research shows that a significant contributor to chronic inflammation comes from what people eat. Many of the foods that are consumed daily worldwide contribute to, or cause inflammation.

Any unhealthy food that is seldom consumed and consumed in small amounts will not cause any harm to the body, but unhealthy foods that are consumed daily will eventually take their toll and cause unhealthy responses in the body, starting with inflammation. Eventually, a continual inflammatory response can potentially lead to weight gain, fatigue, skin problems, problems within the gastrointestinal tract and diseases like diabetes, morbid obesity and cancer.

The Western World has made a radical and ongoing shift towards fast foods and highly processed foods since the 1950's, so to many people, the foods listed below will seem healthy because they are foods that are readily available at grocery stores and supermarkets. They are also the types of food that are prepared and consumed daily in most households. For many people born during the 1960's onwards, these are the only types of food that they know and are comfortable with. Moving away from these foods for many people not only requires a change of diet, but also a change of mindset.

Manufacturers add excessive amounts of unhealthy ingredients to products to enhance the flavors, improve the color and extend the shelf-life with little concern over the health of the consumer. It is not uncommon for manufacturers to disguise unhealthy ingredients by using unusual ingredient names on the printed labels. It is important that consumers take responsibility for their own health by carefully reading the printed nutritional food labels of pre-prepared and processed foods as well as fast foods and not buying foods that contain high amounts of salt and sugar, artificial fats, as well as chemical preservatives, additives, coloring and flavoring. Any food that has unpronounceable ingredients, or ingredients made up of alpha and numeric sequences that do not form a word, printed on the nutritional food label should be avoided and not consumed. These ingredients are most certainly chemicals that should not be consumed and do not belong in the human body. It is always best to completely avoid processed and pre-prepared foods and prepare fresh foods and sauces at home.

The following foods have been clinically proven to promote or cause inflammation in the body. These foods must be avoided and, although sudden total elimination is not always practical or possible, efforts must be made to gradually eliminate them and replace them with healthier alternatives.

- **Sugar**
  When refined and processed sugar is consumed daily and in high amounts, the body is unable to process the excess glucose expediently. This results in increased levels of pro-inflammatory signalling molecules like cytokines in the body. Also, sugar suppresses the effectiveness of white blood cells, placing strain on the immune system. Added sugar can be obvious, or it can be hidden in many fast foods and processed foods. To control sugar intake, it is best to buy only fresh produce and avoid pre-prepared meals, bottled and canned foods and sauces and dehydrated cake, dessert and sauce mixes. There are canned fruit and vegetable products that are free of preservatives, as well as salt and sugar. They generally are more expensive, but they are worth buying over standard bottle and canned products that are packed with preservatives, as well as salt and sugar. Some of the everyday processed foods that contain high levels of sugar include:
  o Energy drinks, energy bars and health bars
  o Soda and fizzy drinks
  o Fruit juice
  o Flavored milk and yoghurt
  o Cakes, sweet pastries, candy and chocolate bars
  o Pre-prepared frozen meals (microwave meals)
  o Pre-prepared sauces and condiments like BBQ sauce, tomato sauce, mustard sauce, as well as salad dressings and marinades
  o Alcoholic and non-alcoholic beverages
  o Flavored and instant breakfast cereals
  o Nut butters

  Health professional worldwide recommend that the maximum amount of added sugars in a daily diet are 37.5 grams or nine teaspoons for men, and 25 grams or six teaspoons for women.

Added sugars can be listed on printed nutritional food labels by different names, including:

- o Anhydrous dextrose
- o Brown sugar
- o Cane juice
- o Confectioner's powdered sugar
- o Corn syrup or corn syrup solids
- o Crystal dextrose
- o Dextrose
- o Evaporated corn sweetener
- o Fructose
- o Fruit nectar
- o Glucose
- o High-Fructose Corn Syrup (HFCS)
- o Invert sugar
- o Lactose
- o Malt syrup
- o Maltose
- o Maple syrup
- o Molasses
- o Raw sugar
- o Sucrose
- o Sugar
- o White granulated sugar

- **Trans fats**
  There are two types of trans fats that are found in everyday food products: naturally-occurring trans fats and artificial trans fats. Naturally-occurring trans fats are produced in the gut of some animals and foods made from these animals may contain small quantities of these fats. Artificial trans fats, also known as trans fatty acids, are produced in a manufacturing process where hydrogen is added to liquid vegetable oils to make them more solid. Artificial trans fats are widely used in fast foods and processed foods, despite clinical studies finding that artificial trans fats are generally not regarded as safe ingredients in human food. The prime reason food manufacturers and food outlets continue to use trans fats is because they are inexpensive, easy to use and extend the shelf-life of products. Trans fats also add flavor and improved texture to food. Many restaurants and fast-food outlets deep-fry foods

in trans fats because oils containing trans fats can be used over and over in commercial fryers before it needs to be discarded.

Trans fats have been proven to raise Low-Density Lipoprotein (LDL) cholesterol levels and lower High-Density Lipoprotein (HDL) cholesterol levels. HDL cholesterol is commonly referred to as good cholesterol, while LDL cholesterol is commonly referred to as bad cholesterol, because it increases the risk of developing heart disease and stroke, promotes inflammation in the body and is associated with a higher risk of developing Type-2 diabetes. Some of the everyday processed foods that contain high levels of artificial trans fats include:

o Baked foods like bagels, cakes, pies, biscuits, cookies, crackers, muffins, pretzels and pizza
o Frozen pie crusts, pizza, pies and sausage rolls
o Dehydrated mixes for cakes, frosting, muffins, waffles, etc.
o Frosting on cakes, biscuits, cookies and doughnuts, as well as cream fillings
o Canned meats and sausages
o Processed cold meats, polonies and sausages
o Fried foods like doughnuts, French fries and any other deep-fried takeaway foods
o Battered or crumbed fish, meat, vegetables, etc. (frozen or takeaway)
o Hard margarine
o Instant flavored noodles
o Ice-cream
o Mayonnaise and salad dressings
o Microwave popcorn
o Non-dairy creamers
o Pre-prepared frozen meals (microwave meals)
o Potato chips and cheese curls
o Pretzels
o Processed meat sticks

Health professionals worldwide recommend that trans fats should be completely eliminated from the diet, as well as all deep-fried foods (the primary source of trans fats in processed and takeaway foods). Check printed nutritional food labels for the ingredients "partially hydrogenated vegetable oils" or "hydrogenated oils" or anything similar and avoid them. Instead look for "0g trans fat" or "un-hydrogenated oil" on printed nutritional food labels.

- **Saturated Fats**
  Regularly eating foods that contain saturated fats does raise cholesterol levels in the blood and high levels of LDL cholesterol increases the risk of developing heart disease and stroke, promotes inflammation in the body and is associated with a higher risk of developing Type-2 diabetes. Saturated fats can be easily identified as any fat that is solid at room temperature. Saturated fats occur naturally in many foods and the majority come mainly from animal proteins, including meat and dairy products. Some of the everyday foods that contain high levels of saturated fats include:

  o All lamb cuts
  o All pork cuts
  o Fat marbled beef
  o Poultry skin
  o Cream and all cheeses
  o Duck fats and similar fats
  o Full cream milk and yoghurt
  o Lard
  o Rendered fat or tallow
  o Coconut oil (does not contain cholesterol)
  o Palm kernel oil (does not contain cholesterol)
  o Palm oil (does not contain cholesterol)
  o Baked and fried foods prepared with any of the above ingredients

  Health professional worldwide recommend that the maximum amount of saturated fats in a healthy daily diet be limited to no more than 5% to 6% of total caloric intake. For example, on a 2,000 calorie (or 8,700 kilojoule) diet per day, saturated fats must not exceed 120 calories (or 522 kilojoules) per day. That equates to about 13 grams of saturated fat per day.

- **Dairy products**
  Probiotics in a limited intake of natural, unflavored yoghurt can

help decrease inflammation in the body, but dairy products are also a source of saturated fats that promote inflammation. Also, clinical studies have linked full-fat dairy products with the negative disruption of gastrointestinal microbiota. This disruption causes a decrease in levels of good gut bacteria that play a major role in reducing inflammation in the body. Dairy products are also a common allergen, with about one in every four adults experiencing some difficulty with digestion after ingesting dairy products. Allergies are mostly due to lactose intolerance or sensitivity in proteins contained in dairy products. All allergens trigger an inflammatory response in the body through the release of histamines. Health professionals worldwide recommend that dairy products be eliminated or greatly limited, particularly in people who suffer from inflammatory conditions.

- **Refined flour**
  Refined wheat flour has been stripped of all slow-digesting fibre and nutrients. Foods made with refined wheat flour are high in glucose and are rapidly broken down in the digestive tract, resulting in a spike in blood sugar levels. The rapid spike in blood sugar levels also causes a spike in insulin levels. A rise in insulin in the blood is directly linked to inflammatory responses in the body. Clinical studies have shown that a diet high in refined grains results in a greater concentration of the inflammatory marker Plasminogen Activator Inhibitor-1 (PAI-1) in the bloodstream. Also, the same clinical studies showed that a diet rich in whole grains resulted in a lower concentration of PAI-1, as well as lower levels of the inflammatory biomarker C-Reactive Protein (CRP). Some of the everyday foods made with refined flour include:

  o Baked foods like bagels, cakes, pies, biscuits, cookies, crackers, muffins, pretzels and pizza
  o Frozen pie crusts, pizza, pies and sausage rolls
  o Battered or crumbed fish, meat, vegetables, etc. (frozen or takeaway)
  o Breakfast cereal
  o Flour tortillas
  o Pasta
  o White bread, white bread rolls and dumplings

Health professionals worldwide recommend that foods made with refined flour should be completely eliminated from the diet and replaced with healthier options. The primary source of foods made with refined flour is convenience, processed and takeaway foods.

- **Artificial sweeteners**
  Clinical studies have found that artificial sweeteners enhance the risk of glucose intolerance by disrupting the balance of the gastrointestinal microbiota. This disruption causes a decrease in levels of good gut bacteria, that play a major role in reducing inflammation in the body. Researchers have also linked glucose intolerance with Type-2 diabetes. When glucose is not metabolized appropriately, it can lead to a greater release of inflammatory cytokines. This inflammatory response is similar to what happens when the body takes in too much sugar and refined flour. Artificial sweeteners are common additives in products labelled as:
  o Diet
  o Low or no calories
  o No sugar added
  o Sugar-free

  Health professionals worldwide recommend that artificial sweeteners should be completely eliminated from the diet and replaced with healthier natural sweeteners.

- **Artificial additives**
  Artificial additives include colorants, flavorings, preservatives and stabilizers. All artificial additives are chemical based and are not fit for human consumption. The digestive system cannot metabolize artificial additives and this can cause from minor irritation in the body to chronic health conditions. Clinical studies have implicated artificial additives in a broad range of conditions from disrupting hormone function to causing hyperactivity, to tumor production. Clinical studies have further shown that the immune system attempts to defend the body from artificial additives and that triggers numerous inflammatory responses in the body. Artificial additives have also been shown to disrupt the balance of the gastrointestinal microbiota, causing digestive and gastrointestinal

complications. Some of the commonly used artificial additives that can be found on printed nutritional food labels include:

- o Acesulfame-potassium (E950)
- o Allura red (E129)
- o Aspartame (E951)
- o Butylated hydroxyanisole (E320)
- o Carmoisine (E122)
- o Carrageenan (E407)
- o Cyclamic acid (E952)
- o Ponceau 4R (E124)
- o Propyl gallate (E310)
- o Quinoline yellow (E104)
- o Sodium benzoate (E211)
- o Sodium nitrite (E250)
- o Sunset yellow (E110)
- o Tartrazine (E102)

Health professionals worldwide recommend that foods containing artificial additives should be completely eliminated from the diet and replaced with natural, healthier options. The primary source of foods containing artificial additives is convenience, processed and takeaway foods.

- **Grain fed meat**
  Grain is not a natural feed for cattle, pigs, sheep or poultry, but the rise of commercial farming that relies on mass production and maximum profits has given rise to feeding livestock and poultry grain. Because a grain-based diet is largely unsuitable, producers have to compensate by administering regular large doses of antibiotics as well. There is little concern shown for the well-being of the animals and birds and none either for the wellbeing of the consumer who will be ingesting the meat and related products. On most commercial farms, livestock and poultry grain are not only administered regular doses of antibiotics, but growth hormones as well, often from birth to slaughter. These drugs prevent disease from spreading in the cramped feedlots and runs, but they also prevent illness from the unnatural diet and greatly speed up unnatural weight gain and growth. The sooner they can get to slaughter, the more profit the commercial farm makes. The other side of this process is that human beings (consumers) are ingesting meat

that is higher in inflammatory saturated fats and has greater levels of inflammatory Omega-6 fatty acids derived from a high corn and soy diet. The result is that a diet high in grain fed meat is going to trigger an inflammatory response. Also, consumers are ingesting remnants of antibiotics and growth hormones, not only in meat products but in all dairy products as well. The added result is that there is a buildup of antibiotics in the body, resulting in a resistance to antibiotic treatment and the buildup of growth hormones can result in an inflammatory response and weight gain.

Health professionals worldwide recommend that meat consumption be limited to three days per week and grain-fed meat be replaced with natural feeds. Organic meat, poultry and dairy products are preferable, because they contain no antibiotics or growth hormones.

- **Processed Meats**
  Processed meats are unhealthy for many of the reasons already mentioned and because they are typically made from red meat cuts, that are high in saturated fats. Processed meats are also Advanced Glycation End Products (AGE's), which are proteins or lipids that become glycated as a result of exposure to sugars dried, smoked, pasteurized, or cooked at high temperatures. These processes create inflammatory compounds that when ingested, trigger an inflammatory response in the body. Many processed meats are also mostly treated with artificial additives. Processed meats include:
  o Bacon
  o Cold meats and polonies
  o Jerky
  o Vienna sausages, hot dogs and various other sausages

  Health professionals worldwide recommend that processed meats should be completely eliminated from the diet and replaced with healthier snacks and options.

- **Alcohol**
  Drinking too much alcohol promotes inflammation in the body. The process of breaking down alcohol in the body generates toxic by-products that can damage liver cells and trigger an inflammatory response, which in turn weakens the body's

immune system. However, the flavonoids and antioxidants in red wine can have an anti-inflammatory effect on the body, if intake is limited to no more than two glasses per day.

Health professionals worldwide recommend that alcohol intake should be moderated to within prescribed limits and should be completely eliminated by people who suffer from inflammatory health conditions.

11.3 Knee Bursitis Eating Plan

Adopting an anti-inflammatory diet will not only help heal knee bursitis and potentially discourage the re-occurrence of the condition, but it will also add value to the quality of life. By cutting back on unhealthy foods that promote inflammation, many other minor health problems, like bloating, fatigue and indigestion, will disappear as will excess weight.

There are many websites and books written by dieticians and health professionals that provide guidance, as well as tasty recipes to make the transition from an unhealthy diet to an anti-inflammatory diet, but for people who are new to the concept, this basic guide is enough to get started. Change is not easy and changing from a diet that has been the norm for years can be intimidating. Adding foreign ingredients and experiencing unfamiliar flavors can make people shy away from the diet change. Therefore, it is best to use familiar ingredients to begin with and experiment with new flavors as the diet changes become more routine.

Anti-Inflammatory Grocery List

The first place to start making diet changes is when shopping for food. That way healthy foods are readily available in the kitchen, making it easier to prepare healthy foods. In the beginning, it is best to buy a range of familiar foods and prepare easy recipes using what is available. As the new anti-inflammatory diet becomes more routine, it will be easier to buy ingredients for specific recipes. An anti-inflammatory grocery list looks similar to this:

- Fresh dark green leafy vegetables like kale, spinach or chard
- Fresh cabbage, cauliflower, broccoli or Brussels sprouts
- Fresh carrots, sweet potato, beetroot, parsnips or turnips
- Fresh salad greens
- Fresh herbs like basil, cilantro or thyme

- Fresh avocados
- Fresh tomato and cucumber
- Fresh onions, leeks, shallots or garlic
- Fresh berries like blueberries, blackberries or strawberries
- Fresh apples, pears, peaches or apricots
- Fresh citrus fruit like oranges, pink grapefruit and red grapefruit
- Fresh ginger
- Fresh chilli peppers
- Pure ground spices like cinnamon, nutmeg, ginger or turmeric
- Pure ground and mixed curry powder
- Dried, canned or frozen beans, legumes or lentils (preservative and sodium free)
- Fatty cold-water fish like anchovies, herring, mackerel, salmon or sardines
- Grass fed (preferably organic) beef, chicken, lamb or pork
- Pure herbal tea
- Dark chocolate (minimum 70%) bars or powder (preferably organic)
- Sprouts, nuts and seeds
- Cold-pressed oils (preferably organic) like canola, extra virgin olive, flaxseed, sunflower or sesame
- Raw oats

Choose fresh, preferably organic, and pure products above processed and pre-packed items, and read the labels carefully. Lemon juice, olive oil or sesame oil, chilli, ginger and salt and pepper make delicious condiments, that can be mixed in a matter of minutes to replace bottles or powdered sauces and salad dressings.

Fresh beans, legumes and lentils are not always readily available. Dried beans, legumes and lentils that are free of preservatives are best, but they do take longer to prepare. Frozen and canned options are also available. Do not choose canned beans, legumes and lentils that come in a sauce like baked beans. These sauces are packed with sugar and artificial additives.

11.4 Recipes to Alleviate Knee Bursitis Pain

While knee bursitis is a physical ailment typically caused by overuse or injury, the foods you eat can have an effect on your level of pain and inflammation. Certain foods have the potential to make your knee bursitis pain worse, while others can help reduce inflammation and relieve pain. To review a bit, here is a list of foods that have been shown to help alleviate bursitis pain:

- Allium vegetables
- Beans and legumes
- Cruciferous vegetables
- Dark, leafy greens
- Hot peppers
- Nuts and seeds
- Root vegetables
- Squashes
- Vegetable sprouts
- Fresh fruits
- Herbs and spices
- Natural oils
- Grass-fed meats
- Eggs and organic poultry
- Cold-water fish
- Green tea
- Dark chocolate

Including as many of these anti-inflammatory foods in your diet as you possibly can is a great way to naturally relieve your knee bursitis pain. These dietary additions can be used in conjunction with conventional treatments for bursitis and they may provide other benefits as well. An anti-inflammatory diet has been associated with numerous health benefits including weight loss, reduced risk for chronic disease, reduced hunger, improved mood, increased energy levels, and more.

If you want to experience the benefits of an anti-inflammatory diet while also alleviating your knee bursitis pain, all you have to do is include more of the foods listed above in your diet. Don't worry – it is easier to do than you think. In fact, you'll find a large collection of anti-inflammatory recipes in this chapter that you can draw from. These recipes are made with fresh, wholesome ingredients from the list provided earlier in this chapter. All you have to do to get started is pick one and give it a try! Here is a list of the recipes you'll find (followed by the actual recipes themselves):

Breakfast Recipes and Smoothies

- Blueberry Banana Smoothie

- Green Tea Overnight Oats
- Broccoli Spinach Frittata
- Pineapple Turmeric Smoothie
- Coconut Chia Breakfast Pudding
- Cinnamon Almond Flour Pancakes
- Ginger Grapefruit Green Smoothie
- Mixed Vegetable Omelet

Lunch Recipes (Soups and Salads)

- Creamy Carrot Ginger Soup
- Balsamic Chicken and Quinoa Bowl
- Hearty Lentil Spinach Soup
- Spinach Salad with Avocado and Almonds
- Fresh Tomato Gazpacho
- Lemon Kale Salad with Toasted Walnuts
- Chunky Beef and Bean Chili
- Southwestern Quinoa Salad Bowl

Dinner Recipes

- Sheet Pan Salmon and Broccoli
- Turmeric Chickpea Balls with Avo-Cream
- Rosemary Roasted Chicken with Veggies
- Sesame Seared Tuna Steaks
- Herb-Crusted Pork Tenderloin
- Seared Scallops with Mango Cream
- Lemon Herb Roasted Turkey Breast
- Grilled Lamb Chops with Chimichurri

Snacks and Dessert Recipes

- Golden Milk Ice Cream
- Turmeric Roasted Chickpeas
- Blueberry Almond Crisp
- Baked Sesame Kale Chips
- Cinnamon Baked Apples
- Coconut Flour Banana Bread
- Avocado Chocolate Mousse
- Honey Mint Fruit Salad

Side Dish Recipes

- Lemon Garlic Sautéed Kale
- Honey-Roasted Carrots
- Simple Sautéed Spinach
- Turmeric Roasted Sweet Potatoes
- Herb Roasted Root Vegetables
- Garlic Cauliflower Mash
- Maple Roasted Brussels Sprouts
- Sautéed Baby Bok Choy

Breakfast Recipes and Smoothies

Blueberry Banana Smoothie

Servings: 1

Ingredients:

- 1 small frozen banana
- 1 cup fresh baby spinach
- ½ cup frozen blueberries
- 1 cup unsweetened almond milk
- 1 tablespoon almond butter
- 1 teaspoon maca powder

Instructions:

1. Combine all of the ingredients in a blender.
2. Pulse several times to chop.
3. Blend on high speed for 30 to 60 seconds until smooth and well combined.
4. Pour into a large glass and enjoy immediately.

Green Tea Overnight Oats

Servings: 2

Ingredients:

- 1 cup old-fashioned oats
- 1 ½ tablespoons chia seeds
- 1 tablespoon hempseed
- ¼ cup cashews, soaked in water for 1 hour
- 1 cup brewed green tea, cooled

- ½ cup unsweetened almond milk
- 1 teaspoon vanilla extract
- ¼ teaspoon ground cinnamon
- 2 pitted dates

Instructions:

1. Combine the oats, chia seeds and hempseed in a bowl.
2. Drain the cashews then transfer them to a blender and add the green tea, almond milk, vanilla, and cinnamon.
3. Pulse several times then add the dates.
4. Blend until smooth and well combined, then pour into the bowl with the oats and stir well.
5. Cover and chill overnight to thicken.
6. Spoon into bowls and top with fresh fruit and nuts to serve.

Broccoli Spinach Frittata

Servings: 6 to 8

Ingredients:

- 8 large eggs
- ½ cup unsweetened almond milk
- 1 clove minced garlic
- Salt and pepper
- 1 tablespoon olive oil
- 1 small yellow onion, diced
- 2 cups fresh chopped broccoli
- ¼ cup water
- 2 cups fresh baby spinach
- ¼ cup sliced green onion

Instructions:

1. Preheat the oven to 425°F (220°C).
2. Whisk together the eggs, almond milk and garlic in a mixing bowl with a pinch of salt and pepper.
3. Heat the oil in a medium cast-iron skillet on medium heat until the oil is shimmering.
4. Add the onion and cook for 5 minutes until translucent.
5. Stir in the broccoli then add the water and cover the skillet – cook for 2 to 3 minutes until the broccoli is bright green.

6. Uncover the skillet then stir in the spinach and cook for 1 minute until it is wilted.
7. Spread the mixture evenly in the skillet then pour in the egg mixture.
8. Season with salt and pepper and sprinkle with green onion then transfer to the preheated oven.
9. Cook for 12 to 15 minutes until just set, then let rest for 10 minutes before slicing to serve.

Pineapple Turmeric Smoothie

Servings: 1

Ingredients:

- 1 ½ cup frozen chopped pineapple
- 1 small navel orange, peeled and chopped
- 1 cup unsweetened coconut water
- 1 tablespoon fresh grated ginger
- 1 teaspoon ground turmeric
- Liquid stevia extract, to taste

Instructions:

1. Combine all of the ingredients in a blender.
2. Pulse several times to chop.
3. Blend on high speed for 30 to 60 seconds until smooth and well combined.
4. Pour into a large glass and enjoy immediately.

Coconut Chia Breakfast Pudding

Servings: 4 to 6

Ingredients:

- 2 cups canned coconut milk
- 1/3 cup unsweetened almond milk
- 1 teaspoon vanilla extract
- ¼ teaspoon ground cinnamon
- Pinch of salt
- ½ cup chia seeds
- Liquid stevia extract, to taste

Instructions:

1. Whisk together the coconut milk, almond milk, vanilla, cinnamon and salt in a mixing bowl.
2. Place the chia seeds in another bowl, then pour the liquid mixture over them.
3. Whisk well and then chill for 20 minutes.
4. Sweeten the pudding to taste with liquid stevia extract, then spoon into bowls or dessert cups.
5. Top with fresh berries to serve.

Cinnamon Almond Flour Pancakes

Servings: 3 to 4

Ingredients:

- 2 large eggs
- ¾ cup unsweetened almond milk
- 1 ½ teaspoons vanilla extract
- 1 ¾ cups almond flour
- 2 tablespoons tapioca flour
- 1 teaspoon baking powder
- Pinch of salt
- 1 tablespoon olive oil

Instructions:

1. Whisk together the eggs, almond milk and vanilla in a bowl.
2. In a separate bowl, whisk together the almond flour, tapioca flour, baking powder and salt.
3. Whisk the dry ingredients into the wet until smooth and well combined.
4. Heat the oil in a large skillet over medium heat.
5. Spoon the batter into the skillet, using about ¼ cup per pancake.
6. Cook until bubbles form on the surface of the batter, then flip the pancakes carefully.
7. Let the pancakes cook until the undersides are browned, then transfer to a plate and repeat with the remaining batter.
8. Serve the pancakes warm with fresh fruit.

Lunch Recipes (Soups and Salads)

Creamy Carrot Ginger Soup

Servings: 4

Ingredients:

- 6 large carrots, peeled and sliced
- 2 medium parsnips, peeled and sliced
- 1 medium yellow onion, chopped
- 6 cloves garlic, minced
- 1 tablespoon olive oil
- Salt and pepper
- 1 teaspoon ground turmeric
- Pinch cayenne
- 6 cups vegetable broth
- ¼ cup fresh lemon juice
- 2 inches fresh ginger, grated
- Unsweetened coconut milk
- Fresh cilantro leaves

Instructions:

1. Preheat the oven to 350°F (180°C) and line a baking sheet with foil.
2. Toss the carrots, parsnips, onion and garlic with the olive oil and spread on the baking sheet.
3. Season with salt and pepper then sprinkle with turmeric and cayenne.
4. Roast for 15 minutes then add to a blender with the vegetable broth, lemon juice and ginger.
5. Blend smooth then pour into bowls.
6. Drizzle with coconut milk and sprinkle with fresh cilantro then serve hot.

Balsamic Chicken and Quinoa Bowl

Servings: 4 to 6

Ingredients:

- 1 cup vegetable stock

- ½ cup uncooked quinoa
- 2 tablespoons fresh lemon juice
- Salt
- 1 tablespoon coconut oil
- 3 tablespoons balsamic vinegar
- 1 teaspoon garlic powder
- 6 boneless chicken thighs, trimmed
- 6 cups fresh chopped romaine lettuce
- 1 ½ cups cherry tomatoes, halved
- ½ medium red onion, diced
- ½ cup fresh parsley leaves

Instructions:

1. Combine the vegetable stock, quinoa, and lemon juice in a small saucepan with a pinch of salt.
2. Bring to a boil then reduce heat and simmer, covered, for 15 minutes until the quinoa absorbs the liquid.
3. Remove from heat and set aside for 2 minutes then fluff with a fork and let cool.
4. Heat the coconut oil in a skillet with the balsamic vinegar and garlic powder.
5. Add the chicken and cook until browned on both sides and cooked through, then remove to a cutting board.
6. Cool the chicken slightly then cut into strips.
7. Combine the lettuce, tomatoes, red onion and parsley in a large salad bowl and toss to combine.
8. Divide the mixture among individual salad bowls.
9. Top with the cooked quinoa and chicken then drizzle with your favorite dressing to serve.

Hearty Lentil Spinach Soup

Servings: 6 to 8

Ingredients:

- 2 tablespoons olive oil
- 1 large yellow onion, chopped
- 3 cloves minced garlic
- Salt and pepper
- ½ tablespoon ground turmeric
- 1 ½ teaspoons ground cumin

- ½ teaspoon ground cinnamon
- 1 (15-ounce or 425grams) can diced tomatoes
- 1 (15-ounce or 425grams) can coconut milk
- ¾ cup dry yellow lentils, rinsed and drained
- 4 cups vegetable broth
- 6 ounces (170grams) fresh baby spinach
- 1 lime, juiced
- Lime wedges

Instructions:

1. Heat the oil in a stockpot over medium heat.
2. Add the onion and garlic then season with salt and pepper – sauté until the onion is translucent, about 5 minutes.
3. Stir in the seasonings and cook for another minute.
4. Add the diced tomatoes, coconut milk, lentils, and broth then season with salt and pepper.
5. Bring to a low boil then reduce heat and simmer, uncovered, for 20 minutes until the lentils are tender.
6. Remove from heat and stir in the spinach until it is wilted.
7. Add the lime juice then adjust seasoning to taste.
8. Spoon into bowls and serve with lime wedges.

Spinach Salad with Avocado and Almonds

Servings: 4

Ingredients:

- 6 cups fresh baby spinach
- 1 cup thinly sliced mushrooms
- ¼ cup thinly sliced red onion
- 3 tablespoons olive oil
- 2 tablespoons fresh lemon juice
- 1 teaspoon Dijon mustard
- Salt and pepper

Instructions:

1. Combine the spinach, mushrooms and red onion in a large salad bowl.
2. Whisk together the olive oil, lemon juice, Dijon mustard, salt and pepper then toss with the salad mix.
3. Divide the salad mix among four plates.

4. Top each salad with sliced avocado and slivered almonds to serve.

Fresh Tomato Gazpacho

Servings: 6 to 8

Ingredients:

- 6 large tomatoes, cored
- 1 cup tomato juice
- 2 tablespoons olive oil
- 1 medium red pepper, cored and diced
- 1 small sweet onion, diced
- 1 seedless cucumber, diced finely
- 1 jalapeno, seeded and minced
- 2 cloves minced garlic
- 2 tablespoons rice vinegar
- ¼ cup fresh chopped cilantro
- Salt and pepper

Instructions:

1. Bring a large pot of water to boil then add the tomatoes.
2. Blanch the tomatoes for about 20 to 30 seconds then transfer to an ice bath using a slotted spoon.
3. When the tomatoes are cool, peel off the skins then cut them in half and remove the seeds.
4. Place the tomatoes in a blender with the tomato juice and olive oil then pulse until pureed.
5. Pour the mixture into a soup serving dish.
6. Add the red pepper, sweet onion, cucumber, jalapeno and garlic.
7. Stir in the rice vinegar and cilantro then season with salt and pepper to taste.
8. Cover and let chill for at least 1 hour before serving.

Lemon Kale Salad with Toasted Walnuts

Servings: 4

Ingredients:

- 2 bunches fresh kale
- ¼ cup olive oil

- 2 tablespoons fresh lemon juice
- ½ teaspoon Dijon mustard
- 1 clove minced garlic
- Salt and pepper
- ¼ cup toasted walnuts, chopped

Instructions:

1. Trim the thick stems from the kale and chop the leaves into bite-sized pieces.
2. Massage the chopped kale by hand for 3 to 4 minutes to get rid of the bitter flavor.
3. Whisk together the olive oil, lemon juice, Dijon mustard, garlic, salt and pepper in a small bowl.
4. Toss the kale with the dressing and divide among plates.
5. Sprinkle with toasted walnuts to serve.

Dinner Recipes

Sheet Pan Salmon and Broccoli

Servings: 4

Ingredients:

- 4 (6-ounce or 170-gram) boneless salmon fillets
- 3 tablespoons olive oil, divided
- Salt and pepper
- 2 cloves minced garlic
- 1 lemon, sliced very thin
- 2 heads broccoli, chopped into florets

Instructions:

1. Preheat the oven to 350°F (180°C) and line a baking sheet with parchment.
2. Place the salmon fillets on the baking sheet and brush with 1 tablespoon olive oil then sprinkle with salt and pepper.
3. Sprinkle the garlic over the salmon fillets and top with slices of lemon.
4. Toss the broccoli with the remaining olive oil and spread on the baking sheet.
5. Season the broccoli with salt and pepper.

6. Bake for 13 to 15 minutes until the fish is just cooked through and the broccoli is tender. Serve hot.

Turmeric Chickpea Balls with Avo-Cream

Servings: 4

Ingredients:

- 1 tablespoon olive oil
- 1 small yellow onion, chopped
- 2 cloves minced garlic
- Salt and pepper
- 1 (15-ounce or 425-gram) can chickpeas, rinsed and drained
- 1 teaspoon ground turmeric
- ½ teaspoon cayenne
- ¼ cup fresh chopped parsley
- ¼ cup almond flour
- 2 small ripe avocados
- Juice from 1 lime
- 2 tablespoons avocado oil
- 2 tablespoons minced red onion
- 2 tablespoons fresh chopped cilantro

Instructions:

1. Heat the oil in a skillet over medium-high heat.
2. Add the onion and garlic and sauté until the onion is browned then remove from heat.
3. Place the chickpeas in a food processor and pulse until it forms a thick paste, scraping down the sides of the bowl as needed.
4. Add the cooked onion and garlic along with the turmeric, cayenne, salt and pepper.
5. Pulse to combine then add the parsley and pulse it into the mix.
6. Shape the chickpea mixture into balls by hand and roll them in almond flour to coat.
7. Reheat the skillet with more oil over medium heat.
8. Add the chickpea balls and cook for 2 to 3 minutes on each side until nicely browned.
9. Combine the remaining ingredients in a food processor and blend smooth then serve with the chickpea balls.

Rosemary Roasted Chicken with Veggies

Servings: 4 to 6

Ingredients:

- 2 tablespoons olive oil
- 2 ½ pounds (1.1 kg) bone-in chicken thighs and drumsticks
- Salt and pepper
- 2 medium sweet potatoes, chopped
- 1 large yellow onion, chopped
- 2 medium carrots, peeled and sliced
- 1 medium parsnip, peeled and sliced
- ¼ cup chicken broth
- 1 tablespoon fresh chopped rosemary
- 1 teaspoon fresh chopped thyme
- 2 cloves minced garlic

Instructions:

1. Preheat the oven to 400°F (200°C).
2. Heat the oil in a large skillet over medium-high heat.
3. Season the chicken with salt and pepper then add it to the skillet – cook for 2 to 3 minutes on each side until browned.
4. Toss the vegetables with the chicken broth, rosemary, thyme and garlic then spread in a large glass baking dish.
5. Place the chicken on top skin-side-down.
6. Roast for 30 minutes then turn the chicken and roast for another 25 to 30 minutes until the juices run clear.
7. Let the chicken rest for 10 minutes then serve hot with the vegetables.

Sesame Seared Tuna Steaks

Servings: 4

Ingredients:

- 1/3 cup black sesame seeds
- 1/3 cup white sesame seeds
- 4 (6-ounce or 180-gram) tuna steaks
- Salt and pepper
- 2 tablespoons olive oil

Instructions:

1. Combine the black and white sesame seeds in a shallow dish.
2. Season the tuna steaks with salt and pepper then dredge in the sesame seed mixture, coating it completely.
3. Heat the oil in a large skillet over high heat.
4. Add the tuna steaks and cook for 1 minute until the sesame seeds on the bottom are golden brown.
5. Turn the tuna steaks and cook for 1 minute on the other side.
6. Transfer to a cutting board and slice thin to serve.

Herb-Crusted Pork Tenderloin

Servings: 8 to 10

Ingredients:

- 1 ½ teaspoons lemon herb seasoning
- 1 teaspoon ground mustard
- Salt and pepper
- 1 (3-pound or 1.4kg) boneless pork tenderloin
- 2 tablespoons olive oil
- 1 tablespoon Dijon mustard
- 1 tablespoon dried basil
- ½ tablespoon dried thyme
- ½ tablespoon dried rosemary
- 1 cup whole-wheat breadcrumbs, plain
- 1 cup dry white wine

Instructions:

1. Preheat the oven to 350°F (180°C).
2. Combine the lemon-herb seasoning, ground mustard, salt and pepper in a small bowl then rub into the skin of the pork tenderloin.
3. Heat the oil in a large skillet over medium-high heat.
4. Add the pork and cook until browned on all sides.
5. Place the pork on a roasting pan and brush with Dijon mustard.
6. Sprinkle with the herbs and breadcrumbs, pressing them into the skin a little bit by hand.
7. Roast for 1 ½ to 1 ¾ hours until the internal temperature reaches 145°F (60°C).
8. Remove the pork to a cutting board and let rest 15 minutes.
9. Stir the wine into the roasting pan, scraping up the browned bits, then pour the mixture into a saucepan.

10. Bring to a boil then simmer until reduced by half.
11. Slice the pork and serve drizzled with the cooking liquid.

Seared Scallops with Mango Cream

Servings:

Ingredients:

- 1 ¼ pounds (600 grams) fresh sea scallops
- Salt and pepper
- 1 ripe mango, chopped
- ¼ cup canned coconut milk
- 1 tablespoon fresh lemon juice
- 1 tablespoon fresh cilantro
- 2 tablespoons olive oil

Instructions:

1. Rinse the scallops in cool water then pat dry with paper towel.
2. Season the scallops with salt and pepper then set them aside while you prepare the mango cream.
3. Combine the chopped mango, coconut milk, lemon juice and cilantro in a food processor and blend smooth.
4. Pour the sauce into a bowl then set aside.
5. Heat the oil in a heavy skillet over high heat.
6. Add the scallops and cook for 90 seconds without disturbing.
7. Carefully turn the scallops and cook for another 90 seconds until just seared in the middle.
8. Transfer the scallops to a paper towel-lined plate to drain.
9. Serve the scallops hot drizzled with the mango cream.

Snacks and Dessert Recipes

Golden Milk Ice Cream

Servings: 8

Ingredients:

- 2 (14-ounce or 400-gram) cans coconut milk
- 1/3 cup powdered erythritol
- 2 teaspoons ground turmeric
- ½ teaspoon ground cinnamon

- ¼ teaspoon ground cardamom
- Pinch black pepper
- 1 teaspoon vanilla extract

Instructions:

1. Combine the coconut milk, powdered erythritol, turmeric, cinnamon, cardamom and pepper in a saucepan.
2. Bring to a simmer then whisk until thoroughly combined.
3. Remove from heat and stir in the vanilla extract.
4. Adjust the seasoning to taste then pour into a large bowl and cool to room temperature.
5. Cover and chill overnight then pour into your ice cream maker.
6. Freeze according to the manufacturer's instructions.

Turmeric Roasted Chickpeas

Servings: 6 to 8

Ingredients:

- 2 (14-ounce or 400-gram) cans chickpeas, rinsed and drained
- 2 tablespoons olive oil
- 1 ½ tablespoons nutritional yeast
- 1 tablespoon ground turmeric
- 1 teaspoon fresh ground pepper
- ¾ teaspoon salt
- ½ teaspoon garlic powder
- Pinch cayenne

Instructions:

1. Preheat the oven to 400°F (200°C) and line a baking sheet with parchment.
2. Toss the chickpeas with the olive oil, nutritional yeast, turmeric, black pepper, salt, garlic powder and cayenne.
3. When evenly coated, spread the chickpeas on the baking sheet.
4. Bake for 60 minutes, stirring every 15 minutes, until crunchy.
5. Turn the oven off and let them cool completely.
6. Store the chickpeas in an airtight container at room temperature.

Blueberry Almond Crisp

Servings: 8

Ingredients:

- 5 cups fresh blueberries
- ¼ cup raw honey
- 2 tablespoon arrowroot powder
- 2 tablespoons fresh lemon juice
- 1 tablespoon fresh lemon zest
- ½ teaspoon ground cinnamon
- 1 cup old-fashioned oats
- ½ cup almond flour
- ½ cup thinly sliced almonds
- ¼ cup coconut sugar
- ¼ cup softened coconut oil
- ¼ cup non-fat Greek yogurt, plain

Instructions:

1. Preheat the oven to 350°F (180°C).
2. Rinse the blueberries well then place them in a square glass baking dish.
3. Stir in the raw honey, arrowroot powder, lemon juice, lemon zest and cinnamon.
4. In a mixing bowl, stir together the oats, almond flour, sliced almonds and coconut sugar.
5. Stir in the coconut oil and yogurt until well combined.
6. Spoon the mixture over the blueberries in the baking dish.
7. Bake for 45 to 55 minutes until the filling is bubbling hot and the topping is just browned.
8. Let the crisp cool for 5 to 10 minutes then serve warm.

Baked Sesame Kale Chips

Servings: 4 to 6

Ingredients:

- 1 large bunch fresh kale
- 2 tablespoons sesame oil
- 1 ½ tablespoons soy sauce
- 1 tablespoon sesame seeds
- Salt to taste

Instructions:

1. Preheat the oven to 300°F (150°C) and line a baking sheet with foil.
2. Thoroughly wash and dry the kale then trim away the thick stems.
3. Cut the leaves into bite-sized pieces and toss them with the oil and soy sauce until evenly coated.
4. Spread the kale on the baking sheet and bake for 10 minutes.
5. Rotate the baking sheet and sprinkle with sesame seeds and salt.
6. Bake for 5 minutes more or until crisp.
7. Remove from the oven and cool completely then store in an airtight container for up to 3 days.

Cinnamon Baked Apples

Servings: 4

Ingredients:

- 4 ripe Granny Smith apples
- 1 tablespoon ground cinnamon
- 1 teaspoon ground nutmeg
- Powdered stevia extract
- Water

Instructions:

1. Preheat the oven to 350°F (180°C).
2. Core the apples and slice them very thin.
3. Place the apples in a glass baking dish and sprinkle with cinnamon and nutmeg then toss to coat.
4. Sweeten to taste with powdered stevia extract then fill the dish about ¼ inch (1 cm) full of water.
5. Bake for 30 minutes until the apples are tender.
6. Spoon the apples into bowls and serve with a drizzle of coconut cream, if desired.

Coconut Flour Banana Bread

Servings: 10 to 12

Ingredients:

- 4 medium bananas, very ripe
- 5 large eggs
- 4 to 5 tablespoons coconut sugar

- 1 teaspoon vanilla extract
- ¾ cup coconut flour
- 1 ¼ teaspoon ground cinnamon
- 1 teaspoon baking soda
- ¼ teaspoon salt

Instructions:

1. Preheat the oven to 350°F (180°C) then grease a loaf pan with coconut oil and line it with parchment paper.
2. Mash the bananas in a bowl then stir in the eggs, coconut sugar and vanilla extract.
3. In a separate bowl, whisk together the coconut flour, cinnamon, baking soda and salt.
4. Whisk the dry ingredients into the wet until smooth and well combined.
5. Spoon the batter into the prepared pan and spread it evenly.
6. Bake for 45 to 55 minutes until the top is firm to the touch and starting to crack.
7. Cool for 15 minutes in the pan then use the parchment paper to lift the loaf out of the pan onto a cooling rack.
8. Let the bread cool completely before slicing to serve.

Side Dish Recipes

Lemon Garlic Sautéed Kale

Servings: 4

Ingredients:

- 2 large bunches fresh kale
- 2 tablespoons coconut oil
- 2 cloves minced garlic
- Salt and pepper
- 2 teaspoons fresh lemon juice

Instructions:

1. Trim the thick stems from the kale then tear the leaves into bite-sized pieces by hand.
2. Rinse the kale well, while bringing a pot of salted water to boil.

3. Add the kale and cook for 4 to 6 minutes until tender then drain and set aside.
4. Heat the coconut oil in a skillet over medium heat.
5. Add the garlic and cook for 1 minute.
6. Stir in the kale and season the mixture to taste with salt and pepper.
7. Cook for 4 to 5 minutes until wilted, then stir in the lemon juice and serve hot.

Honey-Roasted Carrots

Servings: 4 to 6

Ingredients:

- 4 bunches fresh carrots, peeled
- 2 tablespoons coconut oil
- 2 tablespoons honey
- Salt and pepper

Instructions:

1. Preheat the oven to 450°F (230°C) and line a baking sheet with foil.
2. Cut the carrots into large chunks, slicing them on the diagonal.
3. Bring a large pot of salted water to boil and place a steamer basket inside.
4. Add the carrots and steam until just tender, about 5 minutes.
5. Drain the carrots and transfer them to a bowl then toss with the coconut oil, honey, salt and pepper.
6. Spread the carrots on the baking sheet and roast for 25 minutes.
7. Spoon the carrots into a serving bowl and adjust the seasoning to taste.

Simple Sautéed Spinach

Servings: 4

Ingredients:

- 2 tablespoons olive oil
- 1 medium shallot, chopped
- 10 ounces (300 grams) fresh baby spinach
- Salt and pepper

Instructions:

1. Heat the oil in a large skillet over medium heat.
2. Add the shallot and cook for 3 minutes until tender.
3. Stir in the spinach and cook until just wilted, 1 to 2 minutes.
4. Season with salt and pepper to taste and serve hot.

Turmeric Roasted Sweet Potatoes

Servings: 4

Ingredients:

- 3 large sweet potatoes
- 2 tablespoons olive oil
- 2 teaspoons fresh grated turmeric
- ½ teaspoon ground cinnamon
- ½ teaspoon dried rosemary
- ½ teaspoon salt

Instructions:

1. Preheat the oven to 350°F (180°C) and line a baking sheet with parchment paper or foil.
2. Peel the sweet potatoes and cut them into wedges.
3. Spread the sweet potato wedges on the baking sheet and drizzle with olive oil.
4. Sprinkle with turmeric, cinnamon, rosemary and salt then toss until they are evenly coated.
5. Roast for 35 minutes until tender then adjust seasoning to taste.

Herb-Roasted Root Vegetables

Servings: 4 to 6

Ingredients:

- 2 medium sweet potatoes, peeled
- 2 medium carrots, peeled and chopped
- 1 large turnip, peeled and chopped
- 1 large parsnip, peeled and chopped
- 1 large yellow onion, chopped
- 2 tablespoons olive oil
- 3 cloves minced garlic
- 1 teaspoon dried thyme

- 1 teaspoon dried rosemary
- Salt and pepper

Instructions:

1. Preheat the oven to 375°F (190°C).
2. Combine the chopped vegetables in a large bowl.
3. Drizzle with olive oil and sprinkle with garlic, thyme, rosemary, salt and pepper.
4. Toss well to combine.
5. Spread the vegetables on a foil-lined baking sheet.
6. Roast for 30 to 40 minutes, stirring once halfway through, until tender and just browned.
7. Spoon the veggies into a bowl and serve hot

Chapter 12: Websites for Knee Bursitis

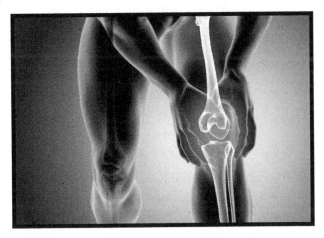

Most valuable resources for knee bursitis are online and to our knowledge there are no books dedicated to knee bursitis on its own other than academic publications.

The following hand-picked online resources offer valuable information, tips and resources for people suffering specifically from knee bursitis.

Equipment

Medical Products and Supplies Online: www.alimed.com

Rally Active Therapeutic Active Wear: www.rallyactive.com

Brace FX: www.bracefx.com

Brace Planet: www.braceplanet.com

All American Supply: www.allamericanmesupply.com

CTi Knee Braces: www.ctikneebraces.co.uk

I On My Braces: www.ionmybraces.com

Kenad Medical: www.kenad.com

Copper Wear Knee: www.copperwearknee.com

Restorative Care of America Incorporated: www.rcai.com

Better Braces: www.betterbraces.com

Zamst Knee Braces and Ankle Compression Socks: www.zamst.us

Sports Braces: www.sportsbraces.com

Leatts Sports Wear: www.leatt.com

Rogue Fitness: www.roguefitness.com

Rehband: www.rehband.com

Very Well Fit: www.verywellfit.com

Tommie Copper: www.tommiecopper.com

RDX Sports: www.rdxsports.com

Strength Shop: www.strengthshop.co.uk

Pod Active: www.podactive.com

Wod Nation Gear: www.wodnationgear.com

Rock Tape: www.rocktape.com.au

Physio Works: https://physioworks.com.

Futuro: https://www.futuro-usa.com

Sport Chek: https://www.sportchek.ca

Rite Aid: https://www.riteaid.com

Galt Tech: http://www.galttech.com

Brace Yourself: https://braceyourself.shop

Treatment Therapies and Exercises

Kris Fondran's Shapeshifter Yoga: https://yogafatlossflow.com

Feel Good Knees: www.feelgoodknees.com

Healthy Self Healing: http://healthyselfhealing.com

Physical Therapy Exercises: https://www.howcast.com

Exercises for Prepatellar Knee Bursitis: https://physioworks.com.au

Alberta Health: https://myhealth.alberta.ca

Knee Bursitis Stretches: https://www.youtube.com

Web MD: https://www.webmd.com

Pharmaceutical Medication

Joint Regen: http://www.asrjointregen.com

Planet Drugs Direct: www.planetdrugsdirect.com

Inicio: www.musicosindependientes.com

Independent Pharmacy: https://www.theindependentpharmacy.co.uk

My Supermarket: http://www.mysupermarket.co.uk

Preparation H: www.preparationh.com

Essential Oils

Bulk Apothecary: www.bulkapothecary.com

Plant Therapy: www.planttherapy.com

Spa Room: www.sparoom.com

CamDenGrey: www.camdengrey.com

Eden Botanicals: www.edenbotanicals.com

Essential Oil: www.essentialoil.com

Essential Oil Labs: www.essentialoillabs.com

Essential Aura: www.essentialaura.com

Goddess of spring: www.goddessofspring.com

Diet and Remedies

Secrets of Turmeric: www.secretsofturmeric.com

Lost Book of Remedies: www.lostbookofremedies.com

Backyard Pharmacy: www.backyardpharmacy.org

Mercola: https://articles.mercola.com

Pinterest: https://www.pinterest.com

Cleveland Clinic: https://my.clevelandclinic.org

Nutritional Living: https://www.nutriliving.com

Kimberly Snyder: https://kimberlysnyder.com

Further Resources

Mayo Clinic: https://www.mayoclinic.org

Medicine Net: https://www.medicinenet.com

American Association of Orthopaedic Surgeons:
https://orthoinfo.aaos.org

Arthritis Health: https://www.arthritis-health.com

Knee And Shoulder Surgery: http://www.kneeandshouldersurgery.com

Chapter 13: Concluding Remarks

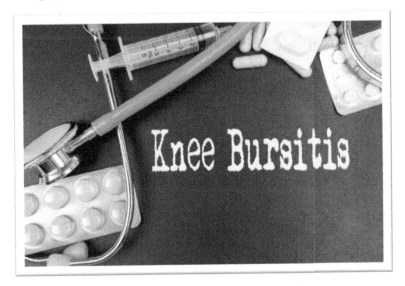

Knee bursitis is inflammation of the bursa cushioning the bones in your knees. Bursa are the fluid-filled sacs that help to reduce friction between moving body parts like your joints. When these sacs become inflamed, it can become incredibly painful – especially with repetitive movements such as walking or climbing stairs.

Though some cases of knee bursitis are mild and resolve on their own, this condition can progress to become very serious and the pain could impact your mobility and your ability to carry out everyday tasks. Fortunately, knee bursitis is fairly easily managed with anti-inflammatory or pain-relieving medications and various therapies or alternative treatments.

In this book, you have learned everything you need to know about knee bursitis and how to treat it. We have walked through the most common types of knee bursitis and their symptoms, as well as treatment options and methods for pain management. You have learned the details of conventional medical treatments as well as alternative therapies, exercises, supplements and even dietary modifications to help reduce or manage your knee bursitis pain. You have also read about helpful exercises to ease your knee bursitis pain and prevent the problem from recurring.

Thank you for buying this book and I sincerely believe and hope that it will help you heal your knee bursitis pain. I have tried to condense all my research findings in this publication to the best of my ability.

Graham Wright, MPhil, Ph.D.

Made in the USA
Middletown, DE
29 September 2021